Composite Tissue Allografts

John Libbey Eurotext
127, avenue de la République
92120 Montrouge
Tél.: 33 (0) 1 46 73 06 60
e-mail: contact@john-libbey-eurotext.fr
http://www.john-libbey-eurotext.fr

John Libbey and Company Ltd
Collier House,
163-169 Brompton Road, Knightsbridge
London SW3 1 PY, England
Tel.: 44 (0) 20 75 81 24 49

CIC Edizioni Internazionali
Corso Trieste 42
00198 Roma, Italia
Tel.: 39 06 841 26 73

© John Libbey Eurotext, 2001
ISBN: 02-7420-0415-7

Illustration de couverture :
© Twice Daily, 2001

All rights reserved. No part of this publication may be reproduced without written permission from the Publisher or the Centre Français du Copyright, 20, rue des Grands-Augustins, 75006 Paris.

Composite Tissue Allografts

CTA 3rd International Symposium
CITIC 2001
29, 30 November 2001

Edited by
Jean-Michel Dubernard

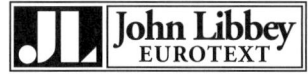

Organizing Committee

P. Cochat

J.-M. Dubernard

J. Traeger

J.-L. Touraine

J.-P. Revillard

C. Dupuy

J.-L. Colpart

V. Lachat

X. Martin

O. Bastien

D. Guillot

International Advisory Committee CITIC

D. Forti *(Milano)*

M. Goldman *(Brussels)*

G.N. Grinyo *(Barcelona)*

P. Lang *(Paris)*

P.J. Morris *(Oxford)*

G. Opelz *(Heidelberg)*

G. Segoloni *(Torino)*

International Advisory Committee CTA

W. Breidenbach *(Louisville)*

N. Hakim *(London)*

M. Lanzetta *(Milano)*

E. Owen *(Sydney)*

Contents

Tribute to Charles Mérieux
J. Traeger XI

Autologous Limb Replantation in Man

Experimental limb transplantation in rodents. Excellent functional recovery and indefinite survival without immunosuppression
M. Lanzetta, C. Ayrout, A. Gal, C. Lauer, E.R. Owen 3

What we have learnt from human hand allograft transplantation
E. Owen, J.-M. Dubernard, M. Lanzetta, N. Hakim, H. Kapila, X. Martin, R. Noli 5

Experimental Data on Composite Tissue Allografts

New trends and future direction of research in composite tissue allotransplantation
F. Petit, A.B. Minns, S.P. Hettiaratchy, D.W. Mathes, J.A. Nazzal, E.R. Svennevik, M.A. Randolph, W.P.A. Lee 9

Immunosuppression in composite tissue allograft
N.S. Hakim 17

Isolated Tissue Allografts in Human

Skin allografts
F. Braye, O. Damour 23

Blood vessels in isolated tissue allografts in man
X. Barral, J.-P. Favre, S. Acquart, S. Chabert 29

Nerve allografts: what is the future?
M. Merle, A. Lim, K. Wieken, G.-B. Lan, C. Bour 35

Ten years follow-up of two cases of vascularized digital flexor system allotransplants
J.-C. Guimberteau 41

Allogeneic vascularized bone and joint transplantation. First five years experience
G.O. Hofmann, M.H. Kirschner 43

Allogeneic hematopoietic stem cell transplantation: current issues and future prospects
G. Socié, E. Gluckman 49

Pathology of the skin after hand allografting
J. Kanitakis, D. Jullien 57

Human Hand Allografts

Hand transplantation: Lyon experience
P. Petruzzo, J.-M. Dubernard 63

The experience of three cases of human hand allografts in China
G. Pei, L. Zhu, L. Gu 69

Immunosupression in hand allograft
N. Lefrançois 71

Bilateral hand transplant: functional results after 18 months
B. Vallet, H. Parmentier, V. Lagouy, N. Dziesmiazkiewiez 75

Cortical reorganisation after hand transplantation
P. Giraux, A. Sirigu, F. Schneider, J.-M. Dubernard 77

Indications for hand allografts
M. Lanzetta 83

The psychiatrist and the hand transplant
D. Bachman, G. Burloux 85

Ethics

Composite tissue allografts: the donor side
D. Houssin, M. Bouvier d'Yvoire, B. Loty 95

Ethical arguments in favor and against the composite tissue allografts
D. Sicard 105

Lecture

Composite tissue allografts: perspectives from a laboratory
W.P. Lee, D.W. Mathes, P.E.M. Butler, M.A. Randolph 111

Contributors

Acquart S., Centre de Transfusion sanguine, Hôpital Bellevue, 42055 Saint-Étienne Cedex 2, France

Ayrout C., Microsearch Foundation Institute, Sydney, Australia

Bachman D., Service de Transplantation, Hôpital Édouard-Herriot, 5, place d'Arsonval, 69437 Lyon Cedex 03, France

Barral X., Service de Chirurgie Cardiovasculaire, Hôpital Nord, 42055 Saint-Étienne Cedex 2, France

Bour C., SOS Mains, Clinique du Pré, 72000 Le Mans, France

Bouvier d'Yvoire M., Établissement Français des Greffes, 5, rue Lacuée, 75012 Paris, France

Braye F., Centre de Traitement des Brûlés, Hôpital Édouard-Herriot, 5, place d'Arsonval, 69437 Lyon Cedex 03, France

Burloux G., Service de Transplantation, Hôpital Édouard-Herriot, 5, place d'Arsonval, 69437 Lyon Cedex 03, France

Butler P.E.M. Plastic Surgery Research Laboratory, Massachusetts General Hospital, Harvard Medical School, Boston MA, USA

Chabert S., Service de Chirurgie Cardiovasculaire, Hôpital Nord, 42055 Saint-Étienne Cedex 2, France

Damour O., Banque de Tissus et Cellules, Hôpital E.-Herriot, 69437 Lyon, France

Dubernard J.-M., Service de Transplantation, Hôpital Édouard-Herriot, 5, place d'Arsonval, 69437 Lyon Cedex 03, France

Dziesmiazkiewiez N., Centre de Val-Rosay, 133, route de Saint-Cyr, 69110 Saint-Didier-au-Mont-d'Or, France

Favre J.-P., Service de Chirurgie Cardiovasculaire, Hôpital Nord, 42055 Saint-Étienne Cedex 2, France

Gal A., Microsearch Foundation Institute, Sydney, Australia

Giraux P., Institute for Cognitive Science, CNRS, 67, boulevard Pinel, 69675 Bron, France

Gluckman E., Service de Greffe de Moelle, Hôpital Saint-Louis, 1, avenue Cl.-Vellefaux, 75475 Paris Cedex 10, France

Gu L., Department of Orthopaedic and Traumatology, Nangfang Hospital, The First Military Medical University, Guangzhou 510515, PR China

Guimberteau J.-C., Institut Aquitain de la Main, 54, rue Huguerie, 33000 Bordeaux, France

Hakim N., Transplant Unit, St Mary's Hospital, 34 Horcraft Road, London NW2 2BL, United Kingdom

Hettiaratchy S.P., Plastic Surgery Research Laboratory, Massachusetts General Hospital, Harvard Medical School, WAC-453, 15 Parkman Street, Boston MA 02114, USA

Hoffman G.O., Berufsgenossenschaftliche Unfallklinik Murnau, Prof. Küntschen Str. 8, D 82418 Murnau, Germany

Houssin D., Établissement Français des Greffes, 5, rue Lacuée, 75012 Paris, France

Jullien D., Service de Dermatologie, Hôpital Édouard-Herriot, 5, place d'Arsonval, 69437 Lyon Cedex 03, France

Kanitakis J., Service de Dermatologie, Hôpital Édouard-Herriot, 5, place d'Arsonval, 69437 Lyon Cedex 03, France

Kapila H., Service de Transplantation, Hôpital Édouard-Herriot, 5, place d'Arsonval, 69437 Lyon Cedex 03, France

Kirschner M.H., Berufsgenossenschaftliche Unfallklinik Murnau, Prof. Küntschen Str. 8, D 82418 Murnau, Germany

Lagouy V., Centre de Val-Rosay, 133, route de Saint-Cyr, 69110 Saint-Didier-au-Mont-d'Or, France

Lan G.B., Institut Européen des Biomatériaux et de Microchirurgie, Université Henri-Poincaré, Nancy I, CHU Brabois, 54500 Vandœuvre-lès-Nancy, France

Lanzetta M., Hand Surgery and Reconstructive Microsurgery Unit, Ospedale S. Gerardo, via Donizetti 106, 20052 Monza, Italia

Lauer C., Microsearch Foundation Institute, Sydney, Australia

Lee W.P.A., Plastic Surgery Research Laboratory, Massachusetts General Hospital, Harvard Medical School, WAC-453, 15 Parkman Street, Boston MA 02114, USA

Lefrançois N., Service de Médecine de Transplantation, Hôpital Édouard-Herriot, 5, place d'Arsonval, 69437 Lyon, France

Lim A., National University Hospital, 5 Lower Kent Ridge, Main Building Level 3, Singapore

Loty B., Établissement Français des Greffes, 5, rue Lacuée, 75012 Paris, France

Martin X., Hôpital Édouard-Herriot, Pavillon V, 5, place d'Arsonval, 69437 Lyon Cedex 03, France

Mathes D.W., Plastic Surgery Research Laboratory, Massachusetts General Hospital, Harvard Medical School, WAC-453, 15 Parkman Street, Boston MA 02114, USA

Merle M., Institut Européen de la Main, 13, rue Blaise-Pascal, 54320 Mexeville, Nancy, France

Minns A.B., Plastic Surgery Research Laboratory, Massachusetts General Hospital, Harvard Medical School, WAC-453, 15 Parkman Street, Boston MA 02114, USA

Nazzal J.A., Plastic Surgery Research Laboratory, Massachusetts General Hospital, Harvard Medical School, WAC-453, 15 Parkman Street, Boston MA 02114, USA

Noli R., University of Milan, Monza, Italy

Owen E.R., Microsearch Foundation Institute, Sydney, Australia

Parmentier H., Hôpital Édouard-Herriot, Pavillon M, 5, place d'Arsonval, 69437 Lyon Cedex 03, France

Pei G., Department of Orthopaedic and Traumatology, Nangfang Hospital, The First Military Medical University, Guangzhou 510515, PR China

Petit F., Service de Chirurgie Plastique, Hôpital Henri-Mondor, 94000 Créteil, France

Petruzzo P., Service de Transplantation, Hôpital Édouard-Herriot, 5, place d'Arsonval, 69437 Lyon Cedex 03, France

Randolph M.A., Plastic Surgery Research Laboratory, Massachusetts General Hospital, Harvard Medical School, WAC-453, 15 Parkman Street, Boston MA 02114, USA

Schneider F., Radiology Department, CHU, 42055 Saint-Étienne Cedex 02, France

Sicard D., Comité Consultatif National d'Éthique, 71, rue Saint-Dominique, 75007 Paris, et Service de Médecine Interne, CHU Cochin, Paris, France

Sirigu A., Institute for Cognitive Science, CNRS, 67, boulevard Pinel, 69675 Bron, France

Socié G., Service de Greffe de Moelle, Hôpital Saint-Louis, 1, avenue Cl.-Vellefaux, 75475 Paris Cedex 10, France

Svennevik E.R., Plastic Surgery Research Laboratory, Massachusetts General Hospital, Harvard Medical School, WAC-453, 15 Parkman Street, Boston MA 02114, USA

Vallet B., Centre de Val-Rosay, 133, route de Saint-Cyr, 69110 Saint-Didier-au-Mont-d'Or, France

Wieken K., Institut Européen de la Main, 13, rue Blaise-Pascal, 54320 Mexeville, Nancy, France

Zhu L., Department of Orthopaedic and Traumatology, Nangfang Hospital, The First Military Medical University, Guangzhou 510515, PR China

Tribute to Charles Mérieux

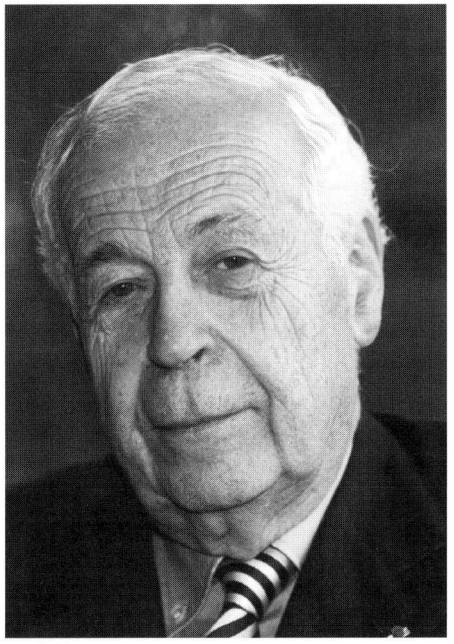

The disappearance of Charles Mérieux marks the close of an exceptionally productive period in the development of human biology; a period where a profound humanitarian mission was backed by a major industrial enterprise.

Charles Mérieux was a true visionary with an extraordinary lucidity in his choices for the future. He knew how to grasp the opportune moment and, after a rapid decision, to move forward decisively. He would then employ patience and tenacity to develop novel ideas and, once his choice was made, he would proceed with calm energy and remarkable perseverance until the success of his project was assured.

This strength of will was backed by a large industrial empire which he had himself built on the basis of the biological laboratory founded by his father, Marcel Mérieux. He had the ability to use the enormous means at his disposal to promote his scientific and humanitarian mission. In 1967 he created the Marcel Mérieux Foundation which supported and promoted numerous projects, meetings, colloquia and symposia, and underwrote research projects and many other activities which sprang from his fertile mind. The many volumes of reports on these activities constitute an exceptionally rich collection.

In this context, Charles Mérieux gave us his unconditional support for the development of the CITIC.

In 1966 we had developed a new type of antilymphocyte serum. With Dr Fries, we had envisaged the use of human thoracic duct lymphocytes as a source of antigen. This material of exceptional purity allowed Dr Carraz of the Lyon Pasteur Institute to immunise his horses under optimal conditions, and to obtain sera with excellent immunosuppressive power and without measurable toxicity. Charles Mérieux immediately realised the importance of this medication, for which he predicted a great future; he was not mistaken because 35 years later it is still used worldwide, particularly in the USA.

From this success grew the idea of an international teaching course on transplantation. The first was held in 1967, and it had been repeated each year since then. No doubt, it satisfied a need growing from the rapid development of transplant medicine and the creation of many new medical teams seeking to implement the technology.

The Mérieux Foundation and its vice president, Mme Claude Lardy, with the assistance of René Triau, then of Caroline Dupuy provided the administrative organisation to ensure the success of the CITIC, as well as the financial support which allowed us to invite top speakers to address the yearly conferences on chosen topics, and to publish a yearly volume of reports.

Dr Charles Mérieux was always present at the opening session of each colloquium. He personally supervised the quality of the programmes presented, even choosing the photographs to be used.

One of Charles Mérieux's attractive qualities was his constant faithfulness to the city where he had established his enterprise, even when it assumed international dimensions. For this reason, and by his express wishes, the CITIC has always remained based in Lyon.

His help for the CITIC was an aspect of his general interest in the development of transplantation technology. This is not the place to list the assistance he provided, but we might mention that in 1972 he supported experimental work in primate xenotransplantation by J.-M. Dubernard, which led, in the same year, to successful human xenotransplantation of chimpanzee kidneys. He also participated in the creation of "Biogreffe" to explore the use of foetal tissue transplantation with J.-L. Touraine, and many years ago he had already organised a bone bank for orthopaedic surgeons.

We all mourn the loss of a man of exceptional humanity. We have lost a friendly mentor who was ever available and ever ready to promote promising new ideas from all sources.

Pr. Jules Traeger
Université Claude-Bernard

Autologous Limb Replantation in Man

Experimental limb transplantation in rodents. Excellent functional recovery and indefinite survival without immunosuppression

Marco Lanzetta, C. Ayrout, A. Gal, C. Lauer, Earl R. Owen
Microsearch Foundation, Sydney, Australia

This study was divided in two parts. Initially, limb transplantation in rats, across the Brown Norway to Fischer 344 histocompatibility barrier, was performed to evaluate the effects of a triple combination immunosuppression therapy and identify the best therapeutic regime. Sixty rats were divided in 5 groups.

Group I consisted of F344 to F344 isografts and Group II allograft controls (BN to F344) receiving no immunosuppressive treatment, whilst Group III-V (BN to F344) received FK506, RS-61443, and prednisolone in different concentrations.

Group III: FK506 0.5 mg/kg/day; RS61443 10 mg/kg/day; prednisolone 0.5 mg/kg/day for two weeks.

Group IV: FK506 2 mg/kg/day; RS61443 15 mg/kg/day prednisolone 0.5 mg/kg/day for two weeks.

Group V: FK506 3 mg/kg/day; RS61443 20 mg/kg/day; prednisolone 0.5 mg/kg/day for two weeks.

At two weeks, in groups III-V prednisolone and RS61443 were simultaneously tapered 20% of the dosage every week; by the 7th week animals were on FK506 only. At this time FK506 was then tapered at the same rate (20% every week) until a maintenance dose of 0.6 mg/kg/day was reached. Evidence of rejection was ascertained by daily visual observation of any swelling, redness, erythema, edema, or skin necrosis. Salvage treatment was used only if rejection occurred after the first 7 weeks. This consisted in reversing to 100% of the initial FK506 dose for that group for 2 weeks, and then tapering was resumed accordingly. Skin and muscle biopsies were obtained from grafted limbs on day 3, 13, 24, 35, and at the endpoint (9 months or uncontrollable rejection).

There was no rejection in Group I, while all animals rejected acutely in Group II as expected. All rats in Group III displayed a similar though delayed acute rejection showing that the chosen regime was not therapeutic. Rats in Group IV displayed the best results, with 10 out of 12 (83%) of them showing no rejection or side effects at the chosen end point of 9 months. Rats in Group V displayed numerous and unacceptable side effects from overtreatment with a mortality rate of 50% at 1 month.

This study showed that low-dose FK506 in combination with RS-61443 and prednisolone can be used to achieve excellent long-term results in case of composite tissue transplantation. FK506 can be used alone as a maintenance therapy following an initial loading dose and a tapering period. Rejection can easily be reversed by increasing temporarily the dose of FK506 only.

In the second part of the study, the three components of our immunosuppressive combination therapy were gradually withdrawn to evaluate the effects on long term survival of the grafted limbs, rejection rate and functional recovery.

The procedure was performed in 8 rats using a strong Brown Norway to Fischer 344 histocompatibility barrier. The animals were given an immunosuppression therapy of FK506 2 mg/kg/day, RS61443 15 mg/kg/day and prednisolone 0.5 mg/kg/day for two weeks. At two weeks, prednisolone and RS61443 were simultaneously tapered 20% of the dosage every week; by week 7 the animals were on FK506 only. FK506 was then tapered at the same rate (20% every week) until a maintenance dose of 0.6 mg/kg/day was reached by week 12.

At 6 months the immunosuppression was stopped; 4 of the 8 animals did not reject throughout the study up to the 1 year end-point. At this stage they showed an excellent functional outcome, evaluated by clinical tests and walking tract analysis. The remaining 4 rats developed a rejection at an average of 267 days postoperatively (range 224-302 days), corresponding to an average of 87 days (range 44-122 days) without any immunosuppression. They were sacrificed for histological examinations of the various tissues.

This study showed that a low-dose triple combination therapy can provide an excellent long term functional outcome of the transplanted limbs, with no rejection episodes, no side effects or complications, even six months after withdrawing of all single components, showing possible tolerance.

Composite Tissue Allografts
Dubernard J.-M., ed.
© John Libbey Eurotext, Paris, 2001

What we have learnt from human hand allograft transplantation

Earl Owen[1], Jean-Michel Dubernard[2], Marco Lanzetta[1,4], Nadey Hakim[3], Hari Kapila[1], Xavier Martin[2], Roberta Noli[4]

[1] *Microsearch Foundation Institute, Sydney Australia*
[2] *Edouard Herriot Hospital, Lyon, France*
[3] *St Mary's Hospital, London, England*
[4] *University of Milan, Monza, Italy*

Following more than a year of success from our first hand allograft on a New Zealander on 23rd September 1998, members of our International Team performed hand allografts on both the hands (simultaneously) of a Frenchman on the 13th January 2000, and on the right hand of an Italian on 22nd October 2000. Follow-up studies range from 12 to 28 months and early conclusions are summarised:

1. Hand transplantation is technically possible both surgically and immunologically.

2. Rejection episodes will occur, as they do in all allografts.

3. But the rejection is seen to begin almost as soon as it occurs in skin.

4. And rejection can be quickly and easily reversed before it becomes established.

5. Monitoring the state of the donor material is easily available.

6. No surgical complications occurred.

7. Rate of nerve regeneration exceeded expectations.

8. Recipients obtained return of protective and useful sensation.

9. Recipients obtained useful function.

10. But function obtained depended upon length of time of forearm atrophy.

11. And functional muscle use also depended upon compliance with exercise regime.

12. Side effects such as minor infections and mild diabetes are transient and controllable.

13. Cerebral cortical re-innovation of wide motor and sensory areas of cortical control reappeared.

14. Current immunosuppressive therapy is effective.

15. And the immunosuppressive drugs can be stepped down in time to low levels.

16. The importance of the patient's prior informed knowledge of the entire procedure and their personality and strict compliance cannot be overstated.
17. The results overall were far more encouraging than those expected in our long pre-planning programme.

The overall **conclusion** is that, with careful case selection, hand allografts will become another routine in the expanding field of transplantation surgery.

Experimental Data on Composite Tissue Allografts

New trends and future direction of research in composite tissue allotransplantation

François Petit*, Alicia B. Minns, Shehan P. Hettiaratchy, David W. Mathes, Jamal A. Nazzal, Eirik R. Svennevik, Mark A. Randolph, W.P. Andrew Lee

Plastic Surgery Research Laboratory, Massachusetts General Hospital, Harvard Medical School, Boston, USA

Composite tissue allotransplantation (CTA) has long been considered a future solution for reconstruction of tissue defects, in which advances in experimental research would one day be made feasible. CTA has now entered the field of human practice and the results of the first procedures performed are encouraging, especially because the prevention of the immunological rejection process is easier than expected [1].

In the past years, immunosuppressive treatments have acquired a high efficacy for preventing acute rejection of organ allografts, and this has also been observed in the recent composite tissue allografts. Seven of 8 hand transplants (uni- or bilateral) performed 1 year ago or more have not been rejected. One hand transplant was rejected 2 years postoperatively after the patient had stopped his immunosuppressive treatment. The prevention of the rejection process currently depends on non-specific immunosuppression that must be high enough to be effective and indefinite, thus challenging the patient with risks of infections, metabolic disorders and malignancy. These side effects are the source of objection for using CTA in reconstructive surgery. Also, current immunosuppressive treatments cannot always prevent the long term functional destruction of some organ allografts, an unfavorable progression called "chronic rejection", with unknown etiology. It is too early to know if composite tissue allografts will be subjected to this phenomenon, but this is a serious threat for the long term functional recovery of these allografts.

Development of allotransplantation for reconstructive surgery depends on our ability to prevent allograft rejection, to obtain a satisfactory functional recovery and to limit the side-effects of therapeutic immunosuppression. Various approaches in research are currently evaluated, and are based on one of the following principles: 1) specific tolerance induction in the recipient by reprogramming or specifically blocking its immune system; 2) genetic matching of the donor and the recipient; 3) development of new drugs and new immunosuppressive protocols. While most of these methods are based on research in organ transplantation, CTA may also benefit from these protocols. However, CTA involves specific constraints due to the nature of the tissue involved, the difficult selection of the grafts, and the need for minimizing the associated morbidity. The nature of CTA justifies the development of specific solutions.

---

* Dr François Petit was supported by a grant from the Philippe Foundation.

Specific tolerance induction

The "holy grail" of researchers in transplantation has always been specific tolerance induction, defined as the absence of the recipient immune response to donor antigens only (presented by the graft). This ideal situation would prevent rejection of the allograft while leaving the recipient fully immunocompetent against other antigens. Specific tolerance induction in the recipient requires interference in the maturation process of T lymphocytes in the thymus or blockage of the activation process of the T lymphocytes encountering the antigen [2].

Hematopoietic chimerism and central tolerance

The most ambitious plan for inducing tolerance is reprogramming the recipient's antigenic repertoire by integrating donor cells. Hematopoietic chimerism can be generated by the addition of donor antigens into the self-repertoire of the recipient. The donor bone marrow derived cells migrate into the recipient's thymus where the presentation of "self" antigens inhibits the release of autoreactive T-cells in the circulation by the clonal deletion or central elimination process [3]. The genetic repertoire of each subject is easily altered during a privileged period of time, prior to maturation [4]. Outside this "window of opportunity", the creation of hematopoietic chimerism requires prior conditioning of the recipient (a destruction of all his/her immunocompetent cells) to allow the engraftment of the donor cells and to prevent their rejection. These conditioning protocols are highly toxic and carry a risk of graft *versus* host disease (GVHD).

Mixed hematopoietic chimerism is achieved with a less toxic conditioning of the recipient *via* the elimination of unnecessary myelosuppression. It results in coexistence of both donor and recipient cells in the recipient's hematopoietic system, thus maintaining a higher immunocompetence of the recipient and reducing the risk of GVHD [5]. The first studies about mixed chimerism were conducted on irradiated mice reconstituted with a combination of donor and recipient bone marrow cells (T-cell depleted) [3]. The mice subsequently received skin allografts, which were accepted when originated from the same donor as the cells but third-party donor allografts were rejected. Later, the use of anti-CD4 and anti-CD8 monoclonal antibodies permitted the reduction in dose of irradiation [6]. In swine, anti-CD3 monoclonal antibodies have been used to deplete the circulating T-cells and thymic irradiation depleted any intrathymic T-cells [7]. Infusion of large numbers of peripheral blood mononuclear cells established a state of mixed chimerism without body irradiation. Kidney allografts from MHC-mismatched swine were accepted without additional immunosuppression [8]. In the cynomolgus monkey, induction of mixed chimerism led to survival of kidney allografts for more than 5 years thus far [9]. Generation of a mixed hematopoietic chimerism has recently been successful to induce tolerance to kidney transplants in humans [10].

Application of mixed chimerism for composite tissue allotransplantation

Our laboratory originally demonstrated the ability to induce a state of mixed hematopoietic chimerism in swine during fetal life (unpublished data). Bone marrow cells from

MHC-mismatched, adult donors were injected into the portal vein under ultrasonic guidance at 50 days (second third) of intra-uterine life. Once born, the swine received a musculoskeletal allograft (limb without skin) from donors identical to the bone marrow cell donors. A 12-day course of cyclosporine was used to prevent rejection due to the minor antigenic differences between the 2 sets of donors. Animals displayed a state of hematopoietic chimerism (1.5 to 26% donor cell chimerism) that led to acceptance of the grafts for more than 250 days without immunosuppression. This study demonstrated that tolerance could be induced for CTA; it was a preliminary step for application to adult recipients. In a study on 13 adult rats, mixed chimerism was induced by injection of a mixture of recipient and donor bone marrow cells (T-cell depleted) along with a short-term treatment with anti-lymphocyte serum and tacrolimus [11]. One year later, limb allografts were transplanted and accepted by the chimeric animals for more than 100 days. Two animals developed GVHD and two animals died from generalized infection. We are currently studying the feasibility of generating mixed chimerism in a large animal model (young adult swine) without prior myeloablation of the recipient. These animals will simultaneously receive an entire limb allograft from fully MHC-mismatched animals. We expect to obtain a prolonged or indefinite survival of the grafts, with no rejection despite the absence of immunosuppression.

Peripheral tolerance and costimulatory blockade

The principle of peripheral tolerance is based on inactivation, or anergy, of circulating T lymphocytes when they encounter the antigen presented by antigen presenting cells. Among the many costimulatory molecules, 4 molecules (CD40/CD154, CD28, B7-1/CD80 and B7-2/CD86) play a major role in initiating the alloimmune response and may be inhibited by 2 selective monoclonal antibodies: anti-CD40-ligand (anti-CD154) and CTLA4-Ig [12]. These agents, while prescribed for the short-term, permitted prolonged survival of heart allografts in rodents and kidney allografts in monkeys, without any other immunosuppressants [13]. So far, these agents could not prevent rejection of skin or limb allografts. Further studies are necessary to assess the efficacy of costimulatory blockade in reducing the overall amount of immunosuppression currently required for CTA.

Donor-recipient genetic matching

Our laboratory described a model of limb allografts between immunologically matched swine (whose major MHC antigens are identical) [14]. In clinical practice, this situation of genetic matching exists between 25% of siblings, but is extremely rare in non-related donor and recipient. Cyclosporine was prescribed for the first 12 days postoperatively only to prevent the rejection due to minor antigens (not identical). Grafts were accepted until the animals were sacrificed (100 to 160 days postoperatively) with no signs of rejection in the osseous, muscular or dermal components of the graft. Skin allografts from mismatched donors (rejected) and from the same donor (prolonged) confirmed that induced tolerance was specific. On the other hand, the tolerance was unsufficient to permit acceptance of the epidermal component of the graft, which was rejected 2 months postoperatively in 3 out of 4 animals [15]. This phenomenon was attributed to the skin immune system and to skin-specific antigens. We now intend to extend our study with this model using a prolonged initial period of immunosuppression and skin-specific (local) immunosuppression of the graft. Clinical application of this situation of tolerance would be a solution in CTA only if a wide registry of genetically pre-identified donors was available.

Advances in therapeutic immunosuppression

New immunosuppressive drugs

Current immunosuppressive drugs may soon be replaced by some of the many new molecules that are currently under experimental evaluation. Sirolimus is the most recent agent that prevents T-cell proliferation by downregulating the activating signal from interleukin-2 (IL-2) [16]. Structurally similar to tacrolimus, sirolimus has a different action, directed at an enzyme called "target of rapamycine" (TOR), which does not prevent IL-2 production, but ultimately inhibits T-cell growth factors. In several phase III studies, when used in human kidney transplantation, sirolimus allowed for the reduction in dose of cyclosporine and withdrawal of steroids. Sirolimus might also reduce lesions of chronic rejection (experimental data). However, blood levels of cholesterol and tryglicerides are usually higher under treatment with sirolimus. Leflunomide inhibits pyrimidine synthesis and, in doing so, prevents lymphocyte proliferation. The first studies on leflunomide for the treatment of rhumatoid arthritis recently resulted in authorization of prescription for patients with this condition. For transplantation, leflunomide prolongs allograft and xenograft survival, and prevents production of anti-donor antibodies (experimental data only). FTY720, a fungal agent, reduces the number of circulating lymphocytes by an unknown mechanism [17]. FTY720 led to prolongation of all kinds of allografts (kidney, heart, liver, skin) in small and large animals. The most prolific field of research on new immunosuppressive drugs is that of anti-T-cell antibodies. Polyclonal antibodies have been used for more than 30 years in the induction phase or to overcome acute rejection of human allografts. Monoclonal antibodies, generated from clonal stem cells in mice (chimeric cells or totally humanized cells), were developed in the recent years. More selective molecules, and therefore less toxic, are currently under experimental evaluation. The association of deoxyspergualine (DSG) with anti-CD3 immunotoxin, a diphteria toxin-derived molecule, could induce donor specific tolerance for renal transplantation on rhesus macaques without episodes of acute rejection or lesions of chronic rejection 1 to 3 years postoperatively [18]. Another antibody, Campath-1-H, directed against the CD52 molecule of the lymphocytes is under clinical trials. One single injection can completely deplete the circulating T and B lymphocytes, and this favors tolerance of the graft [19].

Immunosuppressive combinations

The use of combined immunosuppressive agents in CTA permits the reduction in dose to lower the specific toxicity of each molecule. It is too early to know if the intensity of therapeutic immunosuppression can be decreased in CTA and if the withdrawal of certain drugs is possible. Tacrolimus has a dual immunosuppressive and neuro-regenerative effect that makes it helpful in limb transplants. Steroids bring about anti-œdematous and anti-inflammatory effects on tissue healing that make them particularly useful during the initial phase of CTA. Their withdrawal would be desirable in the long-term, provided that this does not favor the development of lesions of chronic rejection on the graft [20].

Local immunosuppression

Unlike organ transplants, composite tissue allografts may be accessible for local immunosuppression, a solution for reducing the overall amount of systemic immunosuppression and for specifically treating the most antigenic component within the graft-skin. For transplantation, topical immunosupressants have only been used for 2 hand transplant recipients [21], but they are routinely used for the treatment of autoimmune dermatological diseases. Unlike cyclosporine, tacrolimus ointment has a more efficient skin penetration. It could prolong the survival of skin allografts in mice and rats without a systemic effect [22, 23]. Locally delivered tacrolimus specifically acts on antigen presenting, epidermal dendritic cells (CD1a+), which initiate and promote the rejection process of the skin component. It prevents class-II MHC antigen expression by the Langerhans cells [24] and induces profound phenotypic and functional alterations of epidermal dendritic cells [25]. Ultraviolet phototherapy (UVA and UVB) is another approach of specifically treating the cutaneous component of tissue allografts by altering antigen presenting function of the epidermal Langerhans cells [26, 27]. UV modulates the immune system by altering cell membranes, cell-cell interactions, surface antigen expression, and cytokine production. These effects are observed after low doses of irradiation, which do not induce malignant transformation of cutaneous cells. Our laboratory is currently evaluating the efficacy of these protocols of skin-specific immunosuppression (tacrolimus ointment and UV) on the specific model of full limb allotransplantation in swine where the epidermis layer is rejected [15].

Conclusion

The scientific community was split over the justification, benefits, and risks of the first composite tissue allografts. CTA holds a tremendous potential for reconstructive surgery, but its development is currently limited by the risk of complications from the immunosuppressive regimen. Experimental research in transplantation – for organ transplants more than for tissue transplants – is rapidly evolving. In the short term, new molecules will broaden the range of immunosuppressive agents, reduce the toxicity of current drugs, and perhaps prevent the lesions of chronic rejection. In the long term, tolerance induction through a preconditionning regimen of the recipient is the most exciting solution because it would avoid the use of any immunosuppressants.

References

1. Dubernard JM, Owen ER, Lanzetta M, Hakim N. What is happening with hand transplants? *Lancet* 2001; 357: 1711-2.

2. Auchincloss HJ, Sykes M, Sachs DH. Transplantation immunology. In: Paul WE, ed. *Fundamental Immunology*. Philadelphia: Lippincott-Raven, 1999: 1175-235.
3. Ildstad ST, Sachs DH. Reconstitution with syngeneic plus allogeneic or xenogeneic bone marrow leads to specific acceptance of allografts or xenografts. *Nature* 1984; 307: 168-70.
4. Leong LY, Qin S, Cobbold SP, Waldmann H. Classical transplantation tolerance in the adult: the interaction between myeloablation and immunosuppression. *Eur J Immunol* 1992; 22: 2825-30.
5. Sharabi Y, Sachs DH. Mixed chimerism and permanent specific transplantation tolerance induced by a nonlethal preparative regimen. *J Exp Med* 1989; 169: 493-502.
6. Sykes M, Szot GL, Swenson KA, Pearson DA. Induction of high levels of allogeneic hematopoietic reconstitution and donor-specific tolerance without myelosuppressive conditioning. *Nat Med* 1997; 3: 783-7.
7. Huang CA, Yamada K, Murphy MC, Shimizu A, Colvin RB, Neville DM Jr., Sachs DH. In vivo T cell depletion in miniature swine using the swine CD3 immunotoxin, pCD3-CRM9. *Transplantation* 1999; 68: 855-60.
8. Fuchimoto Y, Huang CA, Yamada K, Shimizu A, Kitamura H, Colvin RB, Ferrara V, Murphy MC, Sykes M, White-Scharf M, Neville DM Jr., Sachs DH. Mixed chimerism and tolerance without whole body irradiation in a large animal model. *J Clin Invest* 2000; 105: 1779-89.
9. Kawai T, Poncelet A, Sachs DH, Mauiyyedi S, Boskovic S, Wee SL, Ko DS, Bartholomew A, Kimikawa M, Hong HZ, Abrahamian G, Colvin RB, Cosimi AB. Long-term outcome and alloantibody production in a non-myeloablative regimen for induction of renal allograft tolerance. *Transplantation* 1999; 68: 1767-75.
10. Spitzer TR, Delmonico F, Tolkoff-Rubin N, McAfee S, Sackstein R, Saidman S, Colby C, Sykes M, Sachs DH, Cosimi AB. Combined histocompatibility leukocyte antigen-matched donor bone marrow and renal transplantation for multiple myeloma with end stage renal disease: the induction of allograft tolerance through mixed lymphohematopoietic chimerism. *Transplantation* 1999; 68: 480-4.
11. Foster RD, Fan L, Neipp M, Kaufman C, McCalmont T, Ascher N, Ildstad S, Anthony JP, Niepp M. Donor-specific tolerance induction in composite tissue allografts [corrected; erratum to be published]. *Am J Surg* 1998; 176: 418-21.
12. Larsen CP, Elwood ET, Alexander DZ, Ritchie SC, Hendrix R, Tucker-Burden C, Cho HR, Aruffo A, Hollenbaugh D, Linsley PS, Winn KJ, Pearson TC. Long-term acceptance of skin and cardiac allografts after blocking CD40 and CD28 pathways. *Nature* 1996; 381: 434-8.
13. Kirk AD, Burkly LC, Batty DS, Baumgartner RE, Berning JD, Buchanan K, Fechner JH Jr., Germond RL, Kampen RL, Patterson NB, Swanson SJ, Tadaki DK, TenHoor CN, White L, Knechtle SJ, Harlan DM. Treatment with humanized monoclonal antibody against CD154 prevents acute renal allograft rejection in nonhuman primates. *Nat Med* 1999; 5: 686-93.
14. Lee WP, Rubin JP, Bourget JL, Cober SR, Randolph MA, Nielsen GP, Ierino FL, Sachs DH. Tolerance to limb tissue allografts between swine matched for major histocompatibility complex antigens. *Plast Reconstr Surg* 2001; 107: 1482-90; discussion 1491-2.
15. Mathes DW, Bourget JL, Randolph MA, Solari MG, Wu A, Sachs DH, Lee WP. Tolerance to vascularized musculoskeletal allografts. *Transplant Proc* 2001; 33: 616-7.
16. Katz SM, Hong JC, Kahan BD. New immunosuppressive agents. *Transplant Proc* 2000; 32: 620-1.
17. Kahan BD. FTY720: a new immunosuppressive agent with novel mechanism(s) of action. *Transplant Proc* 1998; 30: 2210-3.
18. Thomas JM, Eckhoff DE, Contreras JL, Lobashevsky AL, Hubbard WJ, Moore JK, Cook WJ, Thomas FT, Neville DM Jr. Durable donor-specific T and B cell tolerance in rhesus macaques induced with peritransplantation anti-CD3 immunotoxin and deoxyspergualin: absence of chronic allograft nephropathy. *Transplantation* 2000; 69: 2497-503.
19. Calne R, Moffatt SD, Friend PJ, Jamieson NV, Bradley JA, Hale G, Firth J, Bradley J, Smith KG, Waldmann H. Campath IH allows low-dose cyclosporine monotherapy in 31 cadaveric renal allograft recipients. *Transplantation* 1999; 68: 1613-6.
20. Morelon E, Kreis H. New immunosuppressive agents: a way to get rid of corticosteroids? *Transplantation* 2000; 70: 1271-2.
21. Francois CG, Breidenbach WC, Maldonado C, Kakoulidis TP, Hodges A, Dubernard JM, Owen E, Pei G, Ren X, Barker JH. Hand transplantation: comparisons and observations of the first four clinical cases. *Microsurgery* 2000; 20: 360-71.
22. Fujita T, Takahashi S, Yagihashi A, Jimbow K, Sato N. Prolonged survival of rat skin allograft by treatment with FK506 ointment. *Transplantation* 1997; 64: 922-5.

23. Yuzawa K, Taniguchi H, Seino K, Otsuka M, Fukao K. Topical immunosuppression in skin grafting with FK506 ointment. *Transplant Proc* 1996; 28: 1387-9.
24. Panhans-Groß A, Novak N, Kraft S, Bieber T. Human epidermal Langerhans' cells are targets for the immunosuppressive macrolide tacrolimus (FK506). *J Allergy Clin Immunol* 2001; 107: 345-52.
25. Wollenberg A, Sharma S, Von Bubnoff D, Geiger E, Haberstok J, Bieber T. Topical tacrolimus (FK506) leads to profound phenotypic and functional alterations of epidermal antigen-presenting dendritic cells in atopic dermatitis. *J Allergy Clin Immunol* 2001; 107: 519-25.
26. Granstein RD, Smith L, Parrish JA. Prolongation of murine skin allograft survival by the systemic effects of 8-methoxypsoralen and long-wave ultraviolet radiation (PUVA). *J Invest Dermatol* 1987; 88: 424-9.
27. Deeg HJ. Ultraviolet irradiation in transplantation biology. Manipulation of immunity and immunogenicity. *Transplantation* 1988; 45: 845-51.

Immunosuppression in composite tissue allograft

Nadey S. Hakim
Transplant Unit, St Mary's Hospital, London, United Kingdom

Composite tissue allografts are non-lifesaving procedures and there is controversy about their use in the reconstruction of large tissue defects. There is obviously concern regarding the potential dangers of lifelong immunosuppression regimes and their accompanying side-effects and risks, which include increased risk of infection, organ toxicity, gastrointestinal toxicity, haematological reactions and increased incidence of cancer and steroid-associated morbidity.

In the last fifteen years, much of the transplant progress has been due to advances in immunosuppressive drugs. A significantly improved understanding of the allo-immune response has allowed for the development of an expanding host of agents that more specifically target the various arms of this immunosuppressive response. At present there are over ten drugs approved by the FDA for clinical immunosuppression, and scores of others are under development.

It is a well known fact that individual tissue components within the composite tissue allograft have differential rejection properties or antigenicity. The skin is considered the most antigenic. The choice of the ideal immunosuppression which would allow graft survival and sensory motor return is the most important factor for the success of this transplant. An important factor why hand transplantation has not advanced as quickly as other organs goes back to the first human case of arm transplant performed in Ecuador in 1964 [1] and in primates during the 1980s [2-4]. At that time immunosuppression was not as advanced as it is today and what was used was azathioprine and hydrocortisone, resulting in complete limb rejection two weeks post operatively.

In the primate studies, cyclosporin was used, suppressing the rejection for a period of up to 296 days [5]. However, the skin portion of the transplanted extremity was rejected within the first month after transplantation. In the primate studies, high dosages of cyclosporin were required and the adverse effects of cyclosporin are well known, nephrotoxicity is the most important and troubling adverse effect. Cyclosporin has a vasoconstrictor effect on the renal vasculature. Long term cyclosporin use may result in interstitial fibrosis of the renal parenchyma, coupled with arteriolar lesions. The exact mechanism is unknown, but renal failure may eventually result. Cyclosporin may also result in a haemolytic syndrome, the clinical features including renal dysfunction, thrombocytopenia and haemolytic anaemia. A number of non-renal side-effects may also be seen with the use of cyclosporin; cosmetic complications, most commonly hirsuitism and gingival hyperplasia, possibly leading to non-compliant behaviour, especially in adolescents and women. A number of neurological complications include headaches, tremor and seizures. Since these early experiences, the new drugs and regimens currently available provide greater protection against rejection while being much less toxic than the previously used drugs. The effectiveness and lower toxicity of these new drugs were demonstrated in pre-clinical animal studies during the mid nineties. Long term limb allograft survival was reported in the porcine composite tissue allograft when using tacrolimus, mycophenolate mofetil (MMF), prednisone combination therapy [6].

Based on this study, the same drug regimens were used in the first successful case of limb transplant, and more hand transplants have been performed since that. Although each team used the same combination of tacrolimus, MMF and prednisone with an induction phase consisting of polyclonal or monoclonal antibodies, there were notable differences in the immunosuppressive regimens used by the different groups. The Lyon and Guangzhou recipients were treated with antithymocyte globulin, whereas the recipient in Louisville received Basiliximab. When looking at the maintenance immunosuppressive regimens, the Guangzhou recipients received much higher doses of prednisone than did the Lyon and Louisville recipients.

Tacrolimus, like cyclosporin, acts by binding immunophylins, its side-effects are similar to those of cyclosporin, most commonly related to nephrotoxicity, neurotoxicity, impaired glucose metabolism, hypertension, infection and gastrointestinal disturbances. It has proven to be of significant benefit in kidney, liver and pancreas transplants. It is superior to cyclosporin for preventing graft rejection and reducing the severity of rejection in liver and pancreas transplants, however there is not enough evidence to suggest that it is superior to cyclosporin in the kidney transplant population.

Polyclonal antibodies directed against lymphocytes have been used in clinical transplantation since 1960. Monoclonal antibody techniques were later developed and in turn allowed for the development of biological agents such as OKT3, which were targeted to specific sub-sets of cells. A number of different monoclonal antibodies are currently under development, many are directed against functionally secreted moleculars of the immune system or their receptors rather than against actual groups of cells.

MMF has got side-effects which are similar to the azathioprine. Notable exceptions are gastrointestinal side-effects which are more common in the MMF group. Clinically important leucopenia is also more common, especially in the higher dose MMF group affecting about one third of the patients. Dose reduction or temporary interruption is usually adequate to treat leucopenia.

Therefore the most controversial question is whether the risks posed by the immunosuppressive drugs justify the benefits. The following complications were reported in hand transplant experiences: tacrolimus-induced or steroid-induced diabetes mellitus requiring insulin therapy; raise in serum creatinine with high dosages of tacrolimus; herpes simplex infection and CMV infections.

The diagnosis of rejection in the hand transplant is easier in view of the unique ability to monitor the rejection by directly observing the skin and performing biopsies in due course and treating accordingly. All rejection episodes encountered in the different centres were diagnosed by performing skin and/or muscle biopsies. Rejection episodes responded to increased dosage of systemic or oral steroids, together with topical application of tacrolimus and clobetasol. Tests used to assess immunological status included flow cytometry, mixed lymphocyte reaction and CD25 typing.

In the first hand allograft performed in Lyon, two acute rejection episodes were detected on days 52 and 77, while in the double hand allograft rejection episodes were encountered at days 57 and 82. In both cases the episodes were completely reversed, increasing the steroid dose and topical application of immunosuppressants. In the first case, chronic rejection lesions such as lichenoid graft *versus* host disease appeared and were treated with anti-CD25 monoclonal antibodies and prednisone. It is interesting to note that in the mixed lymphocyte reaction tests, recipients from Lyon and Louisville showed hyporesponsiveness against the donor and pathogens during the first three months. However at three months both became responsive to both donors and pathogens. The Chinese recipients showed hyporesponsiveness to donor at 8 months post-transplant. There was absence of rejection episodes in both Chinese recipients at 8 months follow-up. The possible explanation for this difference with the other teams' experience is the possibility of having had higher doses of steroids and the better match in those patients compared to the experience seen in the Lyon and Louisville recipients although, with the current immunosuppression, the HLA mismatching has not been as important as it used to be, and it is not known whether it has a special importance in the clinical application of composite tissue allograft. In the Chinese experience, the bone marrow was removed from the donor hands and one of the donors was irradiated. Whether those two extra factors have contributed to the lack of rejection is difficult to confirm. Radiation has been used in the past in the early days of transplantation, especially in the kidney transplantation experience. The donor bone marrow can potentially induce graft *versus* host disease, however no such episodes have been encountered in any of the experiences so far.

In the rat hind limb models, bone marrow has been shown to induce chimerism [7, 8]. Chimerism is the co-existence of both the donor's and the recipient's immune system in the recipient. It has been hoped that the chimerism can itself induce a state of tolerance without the necessity of administering immunosuppressive drugs. However, no chimerism was detected in the patients transplanted in Lyon and Louisville [9].

In conclusion, in hand transplantation we are able to monitor rejection by direct observation of the skin. The most common complications related to immunosuppression are opportunistic infections, which are successfully treated. None of the recipients have so far experienced complications of end organ failure and there were no neoplasms detected. Based on the pre-clinical animal experiments and clinical experiments, tacrolimus based combination is effective at preventing composite tissue allograft rejection.

Should we in the future immunomodulate the donor tissues and pre-treat the donor with new biological agents? Should we perfuse the donor limb with monoclonal antibodies or immunomodulate the donor bone marrow cells to induce donor specific tolerance? Many questions remain unanswered.

References

1. Gilbert R. Transplant is successful with a cadaver forearm. *Med Trib Med News* 1964; 5: 20.

2. Egorszegi EP, Sumulack DD, Daniel RK. Experimental models in primates for reconstructive surgery utilizing tissue transplants. *Ann Plast Surg* 1984; 5: 20.
3. Jones JW, Gruber SA, Barker JH, Breidenbach WC. Successful hand transplantation: one year follow up. *N Engl J Med* 2000: 343: 468-74.
4. Hovins SE, Stevens HP, ven Nierop PW, Rating W, Van Strik R, van der Meulen JC. Allogeneic transplantation of the radial side of the hand in the rhesus monkey: I Technical aspects. *Plast Reconstr Surg* 1992; 89; 700-9.
5. Stark GB, Swartz WM, Narayanan K, Moller AR. Hand transplantation in baboons. *Transplant Proc* 1987; 19: 3968-71.
6. Jones JW, Gruber SA, for Louisville Hand Transplant Research Group. From bench to bedside: porcine extremity composite tissue allograft to human hand transplant. Immunoledge International Meeting, Observer, July 1999.
7. Hewitt CW, Ramsamooj R, Patel MP, Yazdi B, Achauer BM, Black KS. Development of stable mixed Tcell chimerism and transplantation tolerance without immune modulation in recipients of vascularized bone marrow allografts. *Transplantation* 1990; 50; 766-72.
8. Liull R, Murase N, Ye Q, Demetris AI, Fournier V, Starzl TE. Vascularized bone marrow transplantation in rats: evidence for amplification of hematolymphoid chimerism and freedom from graft *versus* host reaction. *Transplant Proc* 1995: 27: 164-5.
9. François CG, Breidenbach WC, Maldonado C, Kakoulidis TP, Dubernard JM, Pei G, Barker J. Hand transplantation: comparisons and observations of the first four clinical cases. *Microsurgery* 2000; 20: 360-71.

Isolated Tissue Allografts in Human

Composite Tissue Allografts
Dubernard J.-M., ed.
© John Libbey Eurotext, Paris, 2001

Skin allografts

Fabienne Braye[1], Odile Damour[2]

[1] Centre de Traitement des Brûlés, Hôpital E.-Herriot, Lyon, France
[2] Banque de Tissus et Cellules, Hôpital E.-Herriot, Lyon, France

Structure of skin

Skin represent a large exposed area, measuring about 18,000 cm^2 for a 65 kg adult. Skin is composed of three different layers, which are, from the surface to the depth, epidermis, dermis and subcutaneous fat.

The epidermis is a cellular membrane, mainly composed with keratinocytes, which progressively differenciate from the basal membrane to form the stratum corneum. Epidermis also contains melanocytes involved in skin pigmentation, Langerhans cells which are responsible for antigens presentation and immune rejection, and Merckel cells which play a role in sensory perception. Epidermis acts as a permeability barrier between the inner and outer environment. Its destruction is life threatening in extensive burns, and its replacement is the main goal of the surgical treatment. In physiological conditions, Langerhans cell free cultured epidermal allografts are rejected and replaced by the keratinocytes of the recipient within 14 days [1].

The dermis is a connective tissue which determines the cosmetic aspect and elasticity of skin. It is mainly composed of a network of collagenous fibers and elastic fibers whose renewal is ensured by fibroblasts. Fibroblasts survive into skin allografts up to 13 months [2].

The subcutaneous tissue is composed of adipocytes. It plays not only the role of an energy storage, but also of a mechanical protection for the underlying structures.

Treatment of burns and skin allografts

In France, about 5,000 persons a year are victims of burns requiring an hospitalisation. Early excision and early closure of the burn wound is the standard of treatment of deep burns. The reconstruction of the epidermal barrier is the main step to achieve wound closure, whereas the replacement of dermis greatly improves the late functional results.

Split thickness autografts from the healthy areas remain the method of choice to achieve the more effective, rapid and cheap coverage. But when burns involve more than 50% of the total body surface, there is not enough healthy skin left on the patient to allow a rapid and definitive skin grafting. Different means of temporary or definitive coverage must then be used [3].

For the treatment of acute burns, the first use of skin allografts was reported by Girdner in 1881 [4]. He initially observed a good engraftment, but at 3 weeks a rejection occurred. Different cases were then reported, but the routine use of allograft for the treatment of burns was clearly described in 1953 [5]. In 1944 Medawar presented a very complete experimental study of skin allografts rejection [6].

Among the different skin substitutes, skin allografts remain the best temporary coverage. Split thickness skin allograft become vascularized and take exactly like an autograft. It then plays the role of a normal skin. For the anesthesiologist, it reduces water, electrolyte and protein loss. It also reduces the energy requirements necessary to the thermal balance and to extensive wound healing. For the local treatment, it prevents burn wound infection and stimulates the vascularization of the wound bed. Wound closure suppresses pain.

After grafting, allografts stay in place between 2 to 4 weeks depending on the immune status of the burned patient. Rejection consists in a progressive loss of the epidermis, while dermis is often incorporated to the burn wound.

All the burn centers agree to say that skin allografts are necessary for the coverage of severe burns [7, 8]. Skin allografts can be used following different techniques, with different goals:

– It can be used as a biological dressing on extensive deep second degree burns. In such burns, deep epidermal appendages are still in place, and provide a reservoir of keratinocytes from which reepithelialization may occur, in optimal conditions. Skin allografts play the role of a biological dressing which prevents surinfection, dessication, and provides growth factors to stimulate wound healing. In such cases, the use of biological dressings or xenografts are good alternatives. Skin allografts can also be used as a temporary skin replacement, after the excision of deep burns. For this application, they are now replaced by xenografts and artificial dermis.

– The association of autograft and allograft, such as the Sandwich technique [9] is an excellent means of coverage. For extensive burns, skin autografts are meshed to increase their surface. When the expansion ratio is greater than 1 to 3, the mesh is very thin and fragile, and most often fails to achieve wound closure alone. In the sandwich technique, skin allografts are applied overlay on the widely meshed autograft, during the same operative procedure. Autograft then progressively develops, under the mechanical and antimicrobial protection provided by allografts, to achieve a complete coverage within a few weeks. This mean of coverage is very efficient, but the limit is the immunological rejection of the allograft within two to three weeks: for the greater expansions of autografts, rejection occurs before the complete closure of the burn wound. For this application, the increase of the survival of skin allografts represents a great interest.

– In the most severe cases, skin allografts are essential for the use of cultured epidermis. The presence of a dermal network is necessary to obtain a good engraftment of cultured keratinocytes. The CUONO technique [10], which is the reference, brings an allogenic dermal bed to cultured epidermis. It lays on an early excision of the burn wound, and an immediate grafting with allografts. When cultured epidermis sheets are ready, about three weeks later, the allogenic epidermis is removed by abrasion. The allogenic dermis stays in place on the patient, and covered with the epidermis sheets. This procedure allows the coverage of very extensive burns over 80% of the total body surface, from a few cm^2 biopsy of healthy skin from the burned patient.

Skin allograft procurement

In France the procurement, conservation and distribution of skin allografts is organized by Tissue Banks and is governed by laws including all the different human tissues [11]. Twenty to 25 m^2 are harvested per year. The evaluation of the surface of allografts required in France is difficult and vary from 50 to 150 m^2 [12]. These variations can be explained by the fact that skin allografts represent the best mean of coverage, and could be used with great benefice for all deep burns, even on less than 50% of the total body. On the other hand, skin is a vehicle for CMV [13] and for HIV [14]. The risk of transmission of known or unknown infectious agents is taken in account to plan skin allografting. Furthermore, the chronic lack of skin allografts results in a economy of this means of coverage. In fact, skin allografts are saved for the more severe patients, presenting life threatening wounds, often over 70% of the total body surface. For such patients, big amounts of allografts are required, and must be replaced when rejection occurs. This is very consuming and uses the skin of several donors for one burned patient. The improvement of the treatment of extensive burns increases survival and subsequently the number of patients requiring skin allografts.

Skin allografts are obtained through three main sources.

– Allogenic skin can be obtained from aesthetic surgery such as abdominal lipectomy. The inconvenient of this method is the small amounts of skin harvested per patients, which results in an expensive multiplication of serological controls. Further more, many skins from different donors are required on the same burned patients, which increases the infectious risk.

– Cadaver skin represents a big reservoir, but the impossibility of late serological controls must be considered. This problem can be solved by using an antiviral treatment of skin such as glycerolization [15].

– Skin from cephalic death allows late serological controls of the organ recipients.

Perspectives

Although research for skin substitutes is a promising perspective for the coverage of burns [3], skin allografts keep necessary for the treatment of the most severe patients. In these conditions, increasing the survival of allografts would be a very significant advance for the treatment of extensive burns at two levels. First, it would improve the yielding of the sandwich technique, allowing huge expansion of the underlying autograft. Secondly, it would avoid the re-applications of allografts on one patient, and subsequently, spare it. To improve the survival of skin allografts, and even to avoid their immunological rejection, two ways of research have been developed; immunosupression of the burned patient or diminution of the antigenicity of the allograft.

The prolongation of life of allografts through an immunosuppression of the burned patient was studied with different immunosuppressive treatments such as azathioprine and antithymocyte globulins [16], cyclosporine [17] or FK506 [18]. Such a treatment increases the susceptibility to bacterial and viral infection, whereas infection is the leading cause of death for these burned patients. This kind of protocol may find a place in the treatment of acute burns when more specific immunosuppression, such as inhibition of interferon α [19], will be achieved.

On the other way, different attemps are made to decrease the immunogenicyty of skin allografts, such as lyophilisation by glycerol [15], incubation in steroids [20], or UVB irradiation [21]. Among these methods, only glycerolization is regularly used, but results in a devitalized allograft with less biological efficiency than living cryopreserved skin.

As a **conclusion**, in spite of their infectious risk, skin allografts remain necessary for the coverage of life-threatening burns. Increasing the number of donors, and if possible delaying their rejection, would represent a great advance for the treatment of extensive burns.

References

1. Aubock J, Irschick E, Romani N, et al. Rejection, after a slightly prolonged survival time, of Langerhans cell-free allogenic cultured epidermis used for wound coverage in humans. *Transplantation* 1988; 45: 730-7.
2. Hull BE, Sher SE, Rosen S, et al. Fibroblasts in isogeneic skin equivalents persist for long periods after grafting. *J Invest Dermatol* 1983; 81: 436-8.
3. Sheridan R, Tompkins RG. Skin substitutes in burns. *Burns* 1999; 25: 97-103.
4. Girdner JH. Skin grafting with grafts from a dead subject. *Med Rec NY* 1888; 20: 119-20.
5. Brown JB, Fryer MP, Randall P, et al. Post mortem homografts as biological dressings for extensive burns and denuded areas. *Ann Surg* 1953; 138: 618-30.
6. Medawar PB. The behaviour and fate of skin autografts and skin homografts in rabbits. *J Anat* 1944; 78: 176-202.
7. Dhennin C. Les allogreffes cutanées: pratiques et souhaits des utilisateurs. Enquête nationale 1995. In: *Brûlures 1997. Actualités de la société française d'étude et de traitement de la brûlure*. Montpellier: Sauraps médical, 1997.
8. Greenleaf G, Hansbrough JF. Current trends in the use of allograft skin for patients with burns and reflexions on the future of skin banking in the United States. *J Burn Care Rehabil* 1994; 15: 428-31.
9. Alexander JW, Mac Millian BG, Law E, Kittur DS. Treatment of severe burns with widely meshed skin autograft and meshed skin allograft overlay. *J Trauma* 1981; 21: 433-8.
10. Cuono C, Langdon R, Birshall N. Composite autologous-allogenic skin replacement: development and clinical applications. *J Invest Dermatol* 1987; 91: 478-85.
11. Pascal P, Damour O, Colpart JJ, Braye F. French legal framework relating to human tissues and cells. *Med Biol Eng Comp* 2000; 38: 241-7.
12. Schlotterer M. Intérêt des allogreffes cutanées dans le traitement des grands brûlés. *Chirurgie* 1997; 122: 6-9.
13. Kealey GP, Aguiar J, Lewis RW, et al. Cadaver skin allografts and transmission of human cytomegalovirus to burn patient. *J Am Coll Surg* 199?; 182: 201-5.
14. Clarke JA. HIV transmission and skin grafts. *Lancet* 1987; 25: 983.
15. Kreis RW, Vloemans AFPM, Hoekstra MJ, et al. The use of non viable glycerol preserved cadaver skin combined with widely expanded autografts in the treatment of extensive third degree burns. *J Trauma* 1989; 29; 51-4.
16. Burke JF, Quinby WC, Bondoc CC, et al. Immunosuppression and temporary skin transplantation in the treatment of massive third degree burns. *Ann Surg* 1975; 182: 183-97.

17. Hewitt CW, Black KS, Achauer BM, et al. Reconstructive allotransplantation: considerations regarding tegumentary musculo-skeletal grafts, cyclosporine, wound coverage in burn injury and the immune response. *J Burn Care Rehabil* 1990; 11: 74-85.
18. Cetinkale O, Cizmeci O, Ayan F, et al. The use of K506 and skin allografting for the treatment of severe burns in an animal model. *Br J Plast Surg* 1993; 46: 410-5.
19. Tovey MG, Benizri E, Gugenheim J, et al. Role of type I interferons in allograft rejection. *J Leukocyte Biol* 1996; 59: 512-7.
20. Alexander JW, Craycraft TK. Prolongation of allogenic skin survival by *in vitro* treatment with fluocinolone acetonide: effect of the incubation time and length of storage. *J Trauma* 1974; 14: 83-0.
21. Alsbjörn BF, Sørensen B. Grafting of burns with widely meshed autograft split skin and Langerhans cell-depressed allograft split skin overlay. *Ann Plast Surg* 1986; 17: 480-4.

Blood vessels in isolated tissue allografts in man

X. Barral[1], J.-P. Favre[1], S. Acquart[2], S. Chabert[1]

[1] Chirurgie cardiovasculaire, Hôpital Nord, Saint-Étienne, France
[2] Centre de Transfusion sanguine, Hôpital Bellevue, Saint-Étienne, France

Arterial allografts were widely used in the 1950s. They were soon abandoned for prosthetic grafts because of low partency rates and frequent anevrysmal degeneration [1]. Since then, tissue preservation techniques have improved with new preservation media and cryopreservation being now available. For these reasons arterial allografts were recently reconsidered, prosthetic graft infection and limb salvage. The aim of this study was to assess long term results of cryopreserved allografts in patients with limb threatening ischemia.

Patients

Between January 92 and December 1999 123 patients underwent 148 by-pass grafts for limb salvage. There were 78 males and 45 females. The mean age was 69.7 years (range 37 to 93 years). The risk factors and major comborbidity were those usually expected in such population: diabete in 54 (48%), hypertension in 70 (57%). The indications for operation were rest pain in 53 patients and major tissu loss in the 70 others. All patients underwent preoperative angiography. In 111 cases (73%) there was at least one previous revascularization and in 48 cases (32%) at least two previous revascularizations. Arterial allograft was indicated in 118 cases because of the absence of greater saphenous vein and in 30 cases because of its unsuitability (dilatation, small size, fibrosis) ABO matching was achieved during the first four years period of the cryopreserved allograft program. Later on, matching was abandoned. In post-op intravenous heparin was administered for 3 days. Antiplatelet drugs and oral anticogulation were subsequently given.

Arterial allograft processing

Arterial allografts were harvested from brain – dead donors as part of the multiple – organ harvesting program. Surgical atraumatic harvesting involved descending thoracic aorta and arteries of the limb from the aortic bifurcation to the tibioperoneal trunk. Cryopreservation was carried out within 20 hours after harvest (4-48H). After a bacteriologic control, arterial allografts were put in freezing bags with dimethyl sulfoxide (DMSO) at 15%. Then, a progressive cryopreservation in a digit cool device with programmed decreasing rate in temperature was performed (cryo Biosystem, l'Aigle, France). The grafts were stored in nitrogen vapor between - 120 ° and 150 °C. A minimal delay of 4 months was allowed before the grafts were used. Thus it was possible to look for seroconversion in recipients of the organs harvested from the same donor. Like wise arterial allografts were discarded in the case of positive bacterial culture. When the use of a cryopreserved arterial allograft was decided, the freezing bag was placed in a water bath at 37 °C to thaw. Grafts were not manipulated until totally thawed to avoid fractures. A new sample for bacterial analysis was performed once the bag was opened. Collateral branches of the graft were ligated with 6-0 polypropylene sutures.

Follow-up

At the begining of the study period in 1992 the twenty first patients have had an invasive follow-up between the third and the six month post-op. Angiography, angioscopy and biopsy under local anesthesia were performed to detect rejection or morphologic changes of the allograft. After this first period conventional follow-up was detected out with duplex scan after the operation at 3.6 and 12 months and yearly thereafter. When the graft was patent, anomalies seen either on duplex scan or angiography were considered to be a failure only if they required an intervention. Cumulative primary and secondary patency, limb salvage and survival rates were assessed with the use of the life table method. Comparaison of estimated was performed with the log-rank test.

Results

Immediate results

During the 30 days post-operative period, the following results were observed:
  – seven patients (5.7%) died. None of these deaths was related to a specific complication of the cryopreserved allograft;
  – two early grafts ruptures were observed at day 21 and day 23;
  – sixteen by-pass occluded after operation requiring subsequent revision, and a total of 10 major amputations. Primary limb salvage at one month was 92.3% Primary and secondary partency rates at one month were 84.8% and 88.9% respectively.

Late results

Mean follow-up was 34.7 months (range 1-93 months). During this period 3 patients (2.4%) were lost to follow-up and fifty eight patient died (47%) *(Figure 1)*.

We observed 84 primary failures (56%): 57 graft occlusions, 10 arterial dilatations, 13 critical stenosis and 4 ruptures; 59 grafts (40%) were surgically revised and 10 grafts occluded again requiring 15 new major amputations. Thus, 25 limbs were amputed in the entire serie.

Primary patency rates at 1.3 and 5 years were 49.8% ± 4.2%, 35; 2 ± 5,6% and 16.9% ± 5.1% *(Figure 2)*.

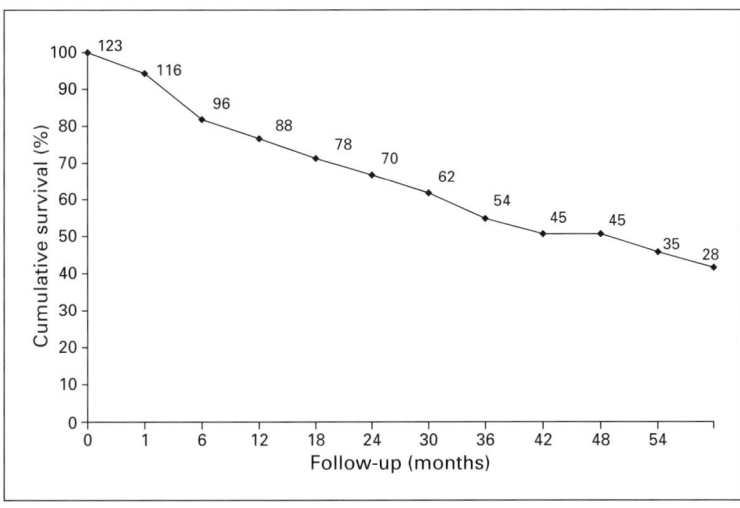

Figure 1. Life-table analysis for survival. Each plot point indicates the number of patients at risk at the beginning of the interval.

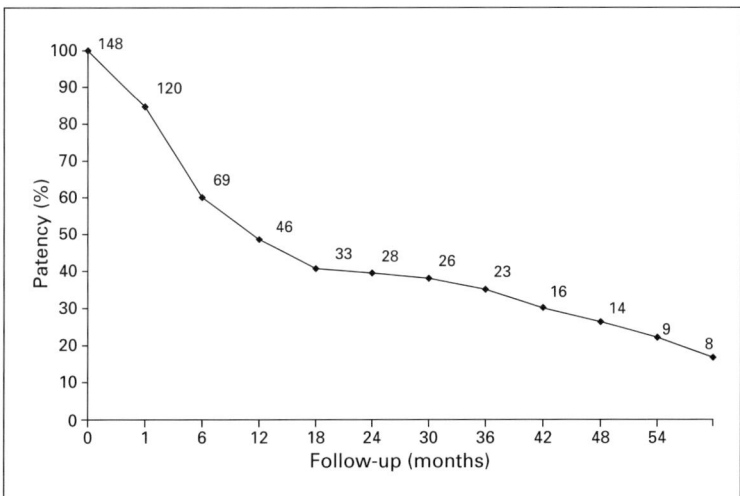

Figure 2. Life-table analysis for primary patency. Each plot point indicates the number of patients at risk at the beginning of the interval.

Secondary patency rates at 1.3 and 5 years were 59.8% ± 4.1%, 45.4% ± 5.9%, 23% ± 5.6% *(Figure 3)*.

Limb salvage rates at 1.3 and 5 years were 82.1% ± 3.6%, 79.5% ± 4.9%; 73.7% ± 6.9% *(Figure 4)*.

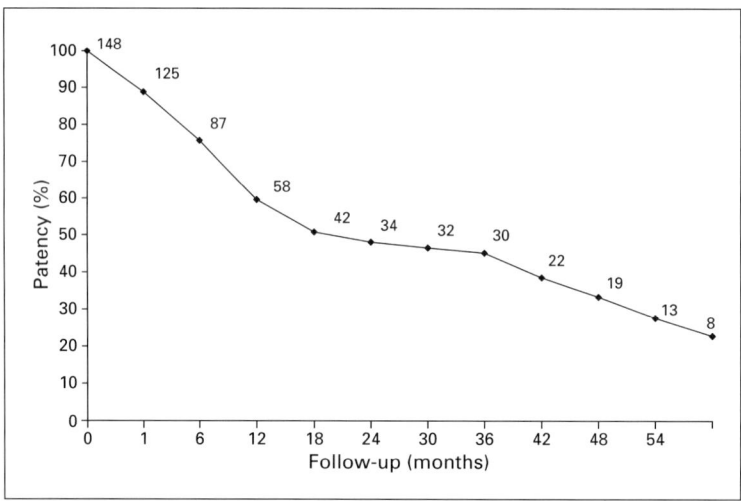

Figure 3. Life-table analysis for secondary patency. Each plot point indicates the number of patients at risk at the beginning of the interval.

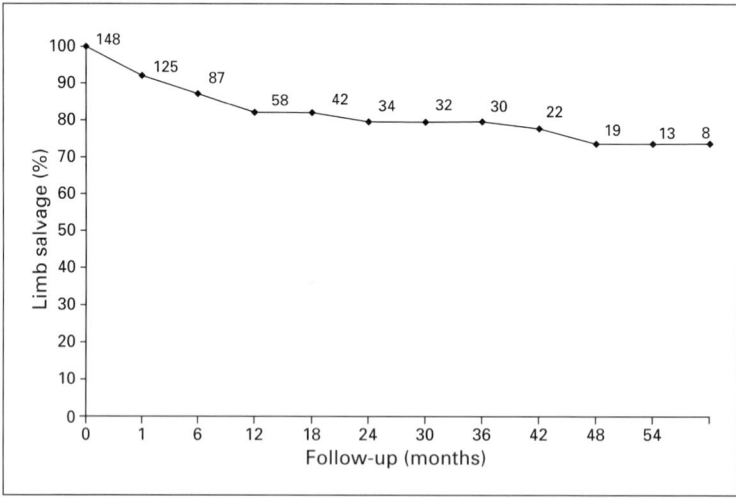

Figure 4. Life-table analysis for limb salvage. Each plot point indicates the number of patients at risk at the beginning of the interval.

Pathologic examination

Thirty-four samples of arterial allografts obtained 3 months ore more after implantation were analyzed. In all cases endothelial and smooth muscle cells were absent with marked medial fibrosis. Lymphomonocytic infiltration was found in only 10 cases.

Discussion

The allograft degradation rate is now lower than reported earlier. Several reasons might explain this difference. New preservation media may cause less damage to arterial allografts than the ones used in 1950. Use of cryoprotectant solution and controlled freezing rate are important improvements that prevent cell damage during freezing. Bench studies have shown the preservation of endothelial and smooth muscle cells properties (contractile activity endothelium dependent and independent relaxation) of arterial allografts after cryopreservation [2, 3]. Nevertheless, incidence of rupture was 4% in this serie with one death. Graft dilatation did not cause death but was responsible for redoprocedures.

In a previous report, we studied the immunological response after arterial allograft. In 20 patients recipient and donor were preoperatively typed for ABO blood group and HLA antigens. All patients had an immunological check-up allowing irregular antibody, allo and auto HLA antibody, antitissu antibody and mixed leucocyte culturs at D0, D21, D5 and D18. Blood groups compatibility have been always matched. On 10 biopsys a polymerase chain reaction (PCR) has been done [4]. At the third month:
– half of the patients (10) have increased HLA antibody of class I or II;
– only recipient cells have been identified in the PCR study. Accorded with histological findings, all these results concorded to demonstrate chronic rejection.

This was confirmed by Plissonier *et al.* They described an early adventicial inflammatory cell infiltration mainly respresented by macrophages and cytotoxic T lymphocytes (CD8) [5]. They have demonstrated the presence of IgG associated with the disappearance of donor endothelial and medial smooth muscle cells. More recently *in vivo*, using allopresentization and aortic allografts they observed an association of allo antibody binding and endothelial cell apoptosis at day 5 and a similar association with smooth muscle cell apoptosis at day 12 [6].

In the same way Mirelli *et al.* [7] have observed that all recipients are likely to develop IgG reactions to donor HLA antigens. This donor specific response is similar to chronic rejection, which occurs in the recipients of vascularized solid organ allografts.

Nevertheless relationship between chronic rejection and patency rate remains unclear. The clinical signifiance of anti HLA antibody in arterial transplant recipients is unknown. In this serie, we observed exactly the same percentage of graft failure (12%) at 6 months between the patients with significant increased HLA antibody class I or II and those without immunological response.

In other respects, in a multicenter study we observed [8] that forty eight percent of late primary failures were due to either progression of distal disease or myointimal hyperplasia, whereas only 15% were due to graft degradation. Therefore, progression of distal disease and myointimal hyperplasia are considered as the two main causes of PTFE graft failure.

Patients were not given immunosuppressive drugs in this series for miscellaneous reasons: old patients with poor general conditions or chronic renal failure, risk of infection in patients with tissue loss. Moreover, in randomized trials, immunosuppressive drugs have failed to improve patency and limb salvage rates with cryopreserved venous allografts [9]. Recently, Mirelli observed no difference in chronic arterial allograft rejection in patients with or without immunosuppresive treatment [7].

Patency rates observed with arterial allografts were clearly worse than those obtained with antogenous saphenous vein. Concerning the comparaison with the PTFE grafts anastomosed on the tibial vessels our opinion is more positive. This serie allowed us to compare two group of patients who were their own witness. 23 of the 148 cryopreserved arterial by-pass concerned femoro tibial grafts performed after the failure of PTFE grafts. They were anastomosed in the same femoro tibial localization. The PTFE graft group had a patency rate of 12% at two years meanwhile the patency rate of the arterial allografts was 36% for the same follow-up period.

There was an important discrepancy between poor late patency and acceptable limb salvage rates. Collateral circulation which developped although the bypass graft was patent, might have provided sufficient blood supply to avoid the recurrence of symptoms when the allograft occluded.

Conclusion

Distal arterial allografts used for distal bypass in patients with critical ischemia lead to acceptable limb salvage but poor patency rates even if they seem better than those observed with PTFE grafts.

Future investigations are to be carried out obtain to better harvesting and better control of the host-grafts interactions.

References

1. Meade JW, Linton RR, Darling RC, et al. Arterial homografts: a long term follow up. *Arch Surg* 1996; 93: 392-9.
2. Rosset E, Friggi A, Novakovitch G, et al. Effects of cryopreservation on the viscoelastic properties of human arteries. *Ann Vasc Surg* 1996; 10: 262-72.
3. Adham M, Gournier JP, Favre JP, et al. Mechanical characteristics of fresh and frozen human descending thoracic aorta. *J Surg Res* 1996; 64: 32-4.
4. Gournier JP, Favre JP, Gay JL, et al. Étude histologique immunologique et clinique des allogreffes artérielles cryopréservées. *Rev Fr Lab* 1996; 280: 65-71.
5. Plissonier D, Nochy D, Poucet P, et al. Sequential immunological targeting of chronic experimental arterial allograft. *Transplantation* 1995; 60: 414.
6. Plissonier D, Henaff M, Poncet P, et al. Involvement of antibody-dependant apoptosis in graft rejection. *Transplantation* 2000; 69: 2601-8.
7. Mirelli M, Stella A, Faggioli GL, et al. Immune response following fresh arterial allograft remplacement for aorto iliac graft infection. *Eur J Vasc Endovasc Surg* 1999; 18: 424-9.
8. Albertini JN, Barral X, Branchereau A, et al. Long term results of arterial allograft below-knee by pass grafts for limb salvage: A retrospective multicenter study. *JV Surgery* 2000; 31: 426-35.
9. Carpenter JP, Tomaszewski JF. Immunosuppression for human saphenous vein allografts by pass surgery: a prospective randomized trial. *J Vasc Surg* 1997; 26: 32-42.

Nerve allografts: what is the future?

Michel Merle[1], Aymeric Lim[2], Karen Wieken[1], Gui-Bei Lan[3], Christian Bour[4]

[1] Institut Européen de la Main, Maxeville, Nancy, France et Institut Européen des Biomatériaux et de Microchirurgie, Université Henri-Poincaré, Nancy I, CHU Brabois, Vandœuvre-lès-Nancy, France
[2] National University Hospital, Singapore
[3] Institut Européen des Biomatériaux et de Microchirurgie, Université Henri-Poincaré, Nancy I, CHU Brabois, Vandœuvre-lès-Nancy, France
[4] SOS Mains, Clinique du Pré, Le Mans, France

The management of gaps in peripheral nerves and brachial plexus injuries made great progress in the 1970s with the concept of interfascicular nerve autografts according to the principles of Millesi [1]. One difficulty however is finding enough grafts and of sufficient length. The promise initially shown by vascularized autografts has been tempered by both the difficulty in finding donor sites with little morbidity and end results comparable with non-vascularized autografts [2].

The successful experience of immunosuppressive treatment for heart, renal, liver and now hand transplants along with extensive experimental evidence plead in favor of using nerve allografts. Freezing grafts and adjuvant immunosuppression allow application of these techniques in humans but there are also unresolved technical and ethical problems, which have limited clinical usage till today.

History

The concept of nerve allografts is not new and it is interesting to note that the clinical case done by Albert in 1885 [3] preceded by 5 years the work of Forsmann [4] who performed a "successful" allograft in a rabbit. This was followed by numerous experimental works till 1945 on dogs, cats and monkeys with results ranging from failure to success.

After 20 years of silence, subsequent work by Das Gupta [5], Zalewski [6], Pollard [7], Chung [8], Comtet [9] and Levinthal [10] between 1967 and 1981 showed constant failure in the rat and pig.

From 1982 onwards, Mackinnon [11], Bain [12], Evans [13] and others demonstrated that nerve allografts in the mouse only work if they are refrigerated in Belzer's solution [14] (University of Wisconsin Cold Storage Solution) for a minimum of 7 days with small doses of cyclosporin A. They also proved that the immunosuppressive effect of monoclonal antibodies prevented rejection of the graft and allowed good regeneration of the nerve [15]. Experimental work was also done in the rabbit and the rat to determine the feasibility of vascularized allografts [16]. In 1985 with C. Bour [17] we evaluated brachial plexus repair in the rabbit and the dog with massive vascularized allograft. These grafts, which were only preserved for a few hours in Ringer's solution before revascularisation, did not undergo any refrigerative treatment. The rabbits were then treated with cyclosporin A and signs of regeneration were obvious during immunosuppressive therapy; however when the treatment was stopped, all the rabbits developed a massive rejection reaction with loss of function. Best, Mackinnon et al. [16] in 1993 compared vascularized autograft and vascularized allograft with and without immunosuppressive therapy in the rat. They proved that vascularized allograft gave equivalent results when compared to vascularized autograft. On the other hand, vascularized allograft without immunosuppression was subject to an acute and massive rejection, with vascular thrombosis possibly accelerated by direct contact with recipient antibodies. Concurrently, we have developed the clinical use of vascularized autografts. However, we realized after a few years follow-up that the functional results were not superior to conventional non-vascularized autografts when the surrounding tissue bed was healthy permitting revascularization of the grafts. The clinical results of vascularized autografts have not been remarkable, which explains the small number of studies on this topic [2].

Experimental data in favor of non-vascularized allografts

Numerous studies mostly done on the rat, rabbit and goat have demonstrated the value of graft pretreatment and adjuvant immunosuppressive treatment with or without monoclonal antibodies.

Pretreatment of grafts

Preservation at 5 °C in Belzer's solution [14] (University of Wisconsin Cold Storage Solution) for a period of 7 days does not diminish the number of Schwann cells but reduces the immunogenicity. Lower doses of cyclosporin are thus required [19, 20]. This period of preservation allows the recipient to be progressively immunosuppressed making allograft nerve grafting an elective operation unlike other allograft procedures. In addition, the number of myelinated fibers during regeneration and the conduction velocity are increased. This effect is particularly evident when FK506 (tacrolimus) is used as the immunosuppressor. Injection of recipient Schwann cells into the allograft also contributes to the protection of the graft from rejection [21].

Immunosuppressive treatments

The benefits of immunosuppression with cyclosporin A have been well demonstrated in the rat [12, 19, 20]. The allograft allows axonal regeneration in the host to proceed. The number of donor Schwann cells diminishes while the recipient Schwann cells colonize the allograft. Without immunosuppression, however, the rejection reaction is very rapid and the allograft becomes a fibrous cord obstructing any nerve regeneration.

Atchabahian *et al.* [22] have demonstrated that immunosuppression can be stopped without detriment to neurological function as long as nerve regeneration has reached the sensory and motor end organs. Generally, at this stage, recipient Schwann cells have finished colonizing the allograft.

Cases of rejection have to be detected early so as to reinforce the immunosuppressive treatment. It is possible to salvage an allograft which is being rejected if FK506 is added within 15 days [23].

Monoclonal antibodies

The usefulness of monoclonal antibodies in anti-rejection therapy for organ transplantation has been well demonstrated. In the rat, different combinations have been shown to protect the allograft from rejection while permitting a decrease in the dose of cyclosporin A. This is the case for ICAM-1, LFA-1 [15] AND CD4 (RIB502) [24]. They are thus useful when there are adverse effects from the immunosuppressive therapy, allowing a decrease in dosages while protecting the graft.

FK506 (tacrolimus) and nerve regeneration

In 1994 Lyons *et al.* [25] showed that in cell cultures, FK506 increases the rate of axonal growth. Since then, numerous studies have confirmed this capability. It has also been reported that weak doses of FK506 on treated allografts allow better functional results in allografts than in autografts [26].

Mackinnon's clinical series [27]

The accumulation of all this experimental data encouraged clinicians to apply the technique of non-vascularized allografts in humans.

S. Mackinnon successfully performed the first case in June 1988, a sciatic nerve to posterior tibial nerve defect in an 11 year old boy was repaired using a 10 strand allograft 23 cm long. After 2 years and two months of immunosuppressive treatment (cyclosporin A), the patient recovered some sensation but no useful motor function. Between 1988 and 1998, Mackinnon carried out 7 allografts on 4 women and 3 men for the following indications: 3 severe median nerve defects, 2 associated with ulnar nerve defects; one radial nerve defect; one sciatic nerve defect and two posterior tibial nerve defects. To facilitate revascularization of the allografts, the nerves were stripped into fascicular groups and all fat was removed. They were also placed under the skin to better monitor for rejection.

The mean age of the subjects was 15 years. The mean length of the allografts was 190 cm. In the first two patients only allograft nerve was used for repair, while the 5 subsequent patients also benefited from autograft sural nerve.

The mean time of immunosuppression was 18 months. Five patients were treated with cyclosporin A and 2 with FK506. Immunosuppression was stopped 6 months after Tinel's sign was detected distal to the allograft with objective signs of return of sensation and muscular function.

The immunosuppressive treatment was:
- cyclosporin A 200 to 300 ng/ml or FK506 5 to 15 ng/ml,
- azathioprine 1 to 1.5 mg/kg/day,
- prednisolone 0.25 to 0.5 mg/kg/day for 5 to 8 weeks.

One graft was rejected after 4 months. The rejection reaction did not however affect the autograft which was partially grafting the ulnar nerve. Long-term follow-up verified a return of protective sensibility in 6 patients, with a two-point discrimination of 3 mm in one patient who had grafting of the ulnar nerve. There was useful motor recovery in 3 cases.

Discussion

Currently, the technique used by all microsurgical teams for repairing nerve defects is interfascicular autografting. Useful functional results, however, rarely occur in more than 60% of the patients of any series [1]. Though vascularized autografts have been useful in large defects, their use is limited by the donor site morbidity and the fact that the functional results are not significantly superior to conventional fascicular autografts [2].

Indications for nerve allografts do exist as shown in Mackinnon's series [27]; in 10 years, she found 10 suitable cases but only seven were operated upon. While the sensory results are encouraging, the motor recovery has been poor but one should note that most of the limbs involved in this series were destined for a total amputation. There are many arguments in favor of allografts; they are certainly an elegant solution for grafting large nerve defects. The problems associated with the immunosuppressive treatment are in part resolved by the limited duration of 18 months on average. Rejection reactions, which do not affect the concurrently placed autografts, are better monitored by placing the grafts subcutaneously. Nervous regeneration definitely benefits from FK506 (tacrolimus) [25].

The main disadvantage is the risk of infection with viruses or even prions. Is it ethical to subject the patient to these risks in the hope of obtaining a purely functional benefit?

Long-term follow-up and a detailed analysis of the secondary effects of the immunosuppressive drugs would clear any ambiguity as to their use.

Even if Mackinnon's experience [27] is unique, she has the great merit of basing her work on a large body of experimental work, systematically resolving all the problems encountered between 1967 and 1981. She was able to overcome them by cold treatment of the grafts for 7 days at 5 degrees. It is also with better immunosuppression protocols and in particular the addition of FK506 that the first clinical cases were possible.

The caution observed by microsurgical teams with regard to allografts will diminish when the principles of allograft nerve regeneration are better known, the adverse effects of immunosuppressive therapy are diminished and the risks of viral or prion infection are addressed.

References

1. Mllesi H, Meissl G, Berger A. The interfascicular nerve grafting of the median and ulnar nerves. *J Bone Joint Surg* 1972; 54A: 727-49.
2. Merle M, Dautel G. Vascularised nerve grafts. *J Hand Surg* 1991; 16B: 483-8.
3. Albert E. Eirige operationen au nerven. *Wien Med Presse* 1885; 26: 1285.
4. Forssman J. Uber den uraschen, welche die wachstrums richtung der peripheren nerven fasern bei der regeneration bestimmern. *Biet Path Anat* 1898; 24: 56.
5. Dos Gupta TK. Mechanism of rejection of peripheral nerve allografts. *Surg Gynecol Obstet* 1967; 125: 1058-68.
6. Zalewski AA. The effect of AgB locus. Compatibility and incompatibility on neuron survival in transplanted sensory ganglia in rats. *Expl Neurol* 1971; 33: 576.
7. Pollard JD, Fitzpatrick L. An ultrastructural comparison of peripheral nerve allografts and autografts. *Acta Neuropathol (Berl)* 1973; 23.
8. Chung PKC, Chung SKY. Evaluation of imuran and locke's solution in peripheral nerve homografts. *Expl Neurol* 1974; 42: 141.
9. Comtet JJ, Revillard JP. Peripheral nerve allografts. Distinctive histological features of nerves degeneration and immunological rejection. *Transplantation* 1979; 28: 103.
10. Levinthal R, Brown J, Ran RW. Fascicular nerve allograft. Evaluation. Part. 1: Comparaison with autografts by light microscopy. *J Neurosurg* 1978; 48: 723-7.
11. Mackinnon SE, Hudson AR, Falk RE, Kline D, Hunter DA. Peripheral nerve allograft: an immunological assessment of pretreatment methods. *J Neurosurg* 1984; 14: 167-71.
12. Bain JR, Mackinnon SE, Hudson AR, Falk RE, Hunter DA. Evaluation of nerve regeneration across nerve allografts in rats immunosuppressed with cyclosporin A. *Surg Forum* 1987; 38: 515-7.
13. Evans PJ, Midha R, Mackinnon SE. The peripheral nerve allograft: a comprehensive review of regeneration and neuroimmunology. *Prog Neurobiol* 1994; 43: 187-233.
14. Evans PJ, Mackinnon SE, Midha R, Wade JA, Hunter DA, Nakao Y, Hare GMT. Regeneration across cold preserved peripheral nerve allografts. *Microsurgery* 1999; 19: 115-27.
15. Nakao Y, Mackinnon SE, Strasberg SR, Hertl MC, Isobe M, Susskind BM, Mohanakuma RT, Hunter DA. Immusuppressive effect of monoclonal antibodies to ICAM 1 and LFA-1 on peripheral nerve allograft in mice. *Microsurgery* 1995; 16: 612-20.
16. Best TJ, Mackinnon SE, Bain JR, Makino A, Evans JE. Verification of a free vascularized nerve graft model in the rat with application to the peripheral nerve allograft. *Plast Reconstr Surg* 1993; 92: 516-25.
17. Bour C, Merle M. Les allogreffes nerveuses et les problèmes immunologiques. *Ann Chir Main* 1989; 8: 334-5.
18. Levi AD, Evans PJ, Mackinnon SE, Bunge RP. Cold storage of peripheral nerves. An *in vitro* assay of cell viability and function. *GLIA* 1994; 10: 121.
19. Mackinnon SE, Midha R, Bain J, Hunter D, Wade J. An assessment of regeneration across nerve allografts in rats receiving short courses of cyclosporin A immunosuppression. *Neurosci* 1992; 46: 585-93.
20. Strasberg SR, Hertl MC, Mackinnon SE, *et al.* Peripheral nerve allograft preservation improves regeneration and decreases systemic cyclosporin A requirements. *Exp Neurol* 1996; 139: 306-16.
21. Ogden MA, Feng FY, Mylkatyn TN, *et al.* Safe injection of cultured schwann cells into peripheral nerve allografts. *Microsurgery* 2000; 20: 314.
22. Atchabahian A, Mackinnon SE, Doolabh VB, Yu S, Hunter DA, Fly MW. Indefinite survival of peripheral nerve allografts after temporaty Cyclosporin A immunosuppression. *Resto Neurol Neurosci* 1998; 13: 129.
23. Feng FY, Ogden MA, Myckatyn TM, *et al.* FK506 rescues peripheral nerve allografts in acute rejection. *J Neurotrauma* 2001; 18: 217.
24. Doolabm VB, Motoyama K, Mackinnon SE, Flye MW. Long term tolerance to peripheral nerve allografts with donor antigen and anti-CD4 monoclonal antibody (RIB 5/2) pretreatment. *Ann Coll Surg Forum* 1998; 49: 633.
25. Lyons WE, George EB, Dawson TM, Steiner JP, Snyder SH. Immunosuppressant FK506 promotes neurite out growth in cultures of PC 12 cells and sensory ganglia. *Proc Natl Acad Sci USA* 1994; 91: 3191.
26. Doolabh VB, Mackinnon SE. FK506 accelerates functional recovery following nerve grafting in a rat nudel. *Plast Reconstr Surg* 1999; 103: 1928.

27. Mackinnon SE, Doolabh VB, Novak CB, Trulock EP. Clinical outcome following nerve allograft transplantation. *Plast Reconstr Surg* 2001; 107: 1419-29.
28. Ansselin AD, Pollard JD, Davey DF. Immunosuppression in nerve allografting is it desirable? *J Neurol Sci* 1992; 112: 160-9.

Ten years follow-up of two cases of vascularized digital flexor system allotransplants

J.-C. Guimberteau
Institut aquitain de la main, Bordeaux, France

The authors have developed for 15 years a series of reconstructive procedures in hand surgery based on island ulnar autotransfers and in particular for tendon repair using the flexor sublimis of the IVth finger and translated forward by a reverse manner able by this way to reconstruct any tendon gap.

In all the cases, they note the excellence of the vascularization of the flexor tendon due largely to small mesovascular pedicle emerging from the ulnar pedicle just before the Guyon's canal.

Moreover, the flexion structures as pulleys, digital canal zone from A1 to A4 are vascularized by collateral vessels coming from the same pedicle, the ulnar vascular system.

This led to the idea of a simultaneous transfer combining tendon and digital canal sheath which are anatomically adjacent, vascularized by the ulnar pedicle in anatomical continuity, in straight line compared to the radial pedicle.

Venous return, potential problem because the small veins beside the artery, has been planed to use the cutaneous vein of the skin ulnar flap which communicates with the superficial veinous network system of the forearm.

Ideas regarding tissue compatibility have evolved over the last few years and the introduction of immunosuppressive drugs efficient with low doses has changed the indications and improved success rates moreover the use of complete flexor tendon system cadaver grafts have been common place in previous years with inconstant results but these experiments reported by E. Peacock have revealed poor antigenicity of collagen tendon structure.

Advances in microsurgical techniques, a better knowledge of the vascularization and pathology of the tendon, with development of antirejection drugs, open new prospects for treatments of repetitive failures, salvage situations and in particular in hand tendons reconstruction.

The use of vascularized tendon allotransplants with a well defined and easily reproducible procedure would seem to be ideal solution.

The advantages are great:
- it is a living transplant, biologically coherent, with an excellent vascularization and intact sliding surface and sliding system;
- it is the exact replica of the original flexion system to be replaced;
- all the tendon sutures are at the wrist, in favourable zones for adhesions;
- the whole procedure is performed in one operating time;
- this procedure can be used for one, two, multiple transfers thanks to the ulnar vascular distribution.

The disadvantages are, of course, the postoperative treatment by immunosuppressive drugs needing a serious blood control and renal tolerance.

But this report of two cases, new type of hand tendon reconstruction, followed by good functional results, reserved at the moment for complex cases, promises future steps if new types of immunosuppressive drugs are set up.

Composite Tissue Allografts
Dubernard J.-M., ed.
© John Libbey Eurotext, Paris, 2001

Allogeneic vascularized bone and joint transplantation. First five years experience

Gunther O. Hofmann, Martin H. Kirschner
Berufsgenossenschaftliche Unfallklinik Murnau, Murnau, Germany

Trauma and infection often result in extended defects of bone and soft-tissues of thigh and knee joint. In many cases the extensor apparatus of the knee joint is usually also affected. In these situations arthroplasty cannot be performed due to technical reasons, if quadriceps tendon and patella ligament are missing. Primary arthrodesis requires subsequent bone-lengthening (Ilizarov's maneuver) to restore the original length of the lower extremity. This procedure is time-consuming, accompanied by a high morbidity and results in various degrees of permanent disability with a stiff leg. Primary above-knee amputation and orthesis is certainly the quickest rehabilitation, but should be considered only as the very last line of defence.

The synthesis of transplant surgery and traumatology created new approaches in these situations. The vascularized allogeneic transplantation of bone and joints may help to restore long-lasting integrity, stability and mobility of the mangled lower leg. In 1990, Chiron *et al.* [1] were the first to report a vascularized allotransplantation of a human femoral diaphysis. In 1994, Doi *et al.* [3] reported a single case of an allogeneic fibula transplanted from a mother to her 2-year-old son. In those procedures no immunosuppression was performed and consequently no revascularization could be detected in the allografted bone. In 1995 our group [4] performed the first clinical vascularized femoral diaphysis allotransplantation employing drug immunosuppression and 1996 the first allogeneic vascularized knee joint transplantation followed [5, 6].

Patients and methods

Until now we have performed vascularized femoral diaphysis allotransplants in three patients and vascularized knee joint allotransplants in five patients. Indications were extensive bone loss after post-traumatic osteomyelitis (n = 2) and chondrosarcoma grade 1 without recurrence for three years (n = 1) in the femoral transplantation and post-traumatic loss of soft-tissues and bone that resulted in defects of 10-15 centimeters in the distal femur and 5-10 centimeters in the proximal tibia in the knee transplant cases. In all 5 patients the extensor apparatus was destroyed. A standardized preparation procedure was established and used in all our transplant cases. After extensive resection of non-viable bone and soft-tissue the defect area was surgically debrided, jet-irrigated and vacuum wound dressing was employed until three consecutive microbiological cultures demonstrated that the defect was free of bacteriological contamination. Local or free flaps were then used to achieve soft-tissue coverage converting the defect into a closed, aseptic cavity.

Femoral diaphysis and knee joints were harvested in accordance with standard organ procurement guidelines used in multi-organ donation. Patients older than 45 years or those who had an accident involving the joint intended for transplant were excluded. After preparation of the abdominal organs, the corresponding external iliac artery was canulated and the leg perfused separately with 4 l of University of Wisconsin solution at 4 °C. Femoral artery and vein were dissected distally to the proximal level of the adductor cannel. The muscles were divided and the femur and tibia were sawed, leaving approximately 5 centimeters of extra length. Particular care was taken not to endanger the vascular pedicle. The harvested graft was stored in sterile conditions at 4 °C. Cold ischemia time ranged from 18-25 hours.

The surgical procedure of the transplantation consisted of five steps. At first, all temporary spacers were removed from the cavities. Another surgical debridement and jet-lavage irrigation of the defects was performed. In the second steps the recipients femoral artery and vein and in cases of knee joint transplantation also the peroneal and tibial nerves were exposed. Under radiographic control the grafts were cut during the third step to the precise size of the defect and put in place. All osteosynthesis were performed with intramedullary interlocking compression nails. In the first step the graft vessels were anastomosed to the recipient's femoral artery and vein using end-to-side technique and the reperfusion of the grafts was started immediately. During the fifth and last step of the procedure the bone grafts quadriceps tendon was inserted into the quadriceps muscle of the recipient of the knee joints.

ABO-compatible grafts were used without matching the HLA status. Crossmatching was done before transplantation and had to be negative. Immunosuppression started immediately after reperfusion of the graft's initially employing four drugs by an intravenous application route: cyclosporine A (1,5 mg/kg daily), azathioprine (1,5 mg/kg BW daily), methylprednisolone (250 mg daily) and anti-thymocyte-globulin (4 mg/kg daily). After the first week the immunosuppressive protocol was switched to an oral double drug maintenance therapy that lasted for the subsequent six months: cyclosporine A (6,0 mg/kg BW p.o.) and azathioprine (3,0 mg/kg BW p.o.). The immunosuppressive maintenance regimen after the first six months consisted of cyclosporine A monotherapy. The post-operative patients that received transplanted femur grafts were mobilized on the first post-operative day. They were allowed to walk immediately with pain-adapted weight bearing. The knee joint recipients were not allowed to bear weight on the transplants during the first three post-operative days. Partial weight bearing increased subsequently and full weight bearing was achieved between six and fifteen weeks after transplantation. All patients were discharged from the hospital between three and eight weeks after transplantation.

The post-operative monitoring of the transplantation consisted of clinical controls (local rejection or inflammation signs, fever) and daily laboratory controls of white blood cell counts, C-reactive proteins, CsA blood levels and PTT. Osseous consolidation of the osteotomies, the position of the nails and screws as well as bone healing was followed by radiographs. Digital subtraction angiograms (DSA) were used to monitor the macroscopic circulation in the graft's pedicle during the first post-operative days and whenever clinical problems occurred. Additionally, duplex sonograms were taken whenever possible during the follow-up. 99m-Tc-DPD scintigraphy was used to assess microcirculatory perfusion and cellular metabolism of the transplanted bone. In case of rejection episodes arthroscopy was performed to examine the joint and biopsy specimens were taken for histological monitoring of cellular perivascular infiltration and viability of cells in the synovial tissue.

Results

Preliminary outcomes of our clinical femoral diaphysis and whole-knee joint allotransplants have been published in detail elsewhere [7, 8]. In all three of our femur diaphysis allograft recipients, the osteotomies showed osseous consolidation within one or two years. In all cases immunosuppression was stopped when X-rays showed bone union of the osteotomies. In two patients, the femoral nails were removed within two years after transplantation. In one patient, an additional total knee arthroplasty, distal to the femoral transplant, had to be performed due to the subsequent development of severe post-traumatic gonarthrosis. In this case the nail was left *in situ*.

Four out of five patients with knee joint allografts were discharged from the hospital four to eight weeks after transplantation. At that time they were mobile and partially weight bearing. Full weight bearing was achieved two to four weeks later. Osseous consolidation of the osteotomy could be demonstrated on X-rays.

In one patient the site of the defect with the allograft became reinfected under the immunosuppressive therapy within the first week post-transplant. In spite of antibiotic therapy, reduction in the dose of immunosuppression and aggressive surgical debridement and lavage of the operative site every second day the infection persisted and urged us to discontinue immunosuppression and remove the allograft. This patient is on her way to arthrodesis employing segment transport procedure.

Meanwhile the other four patients all have received additional total knee arthroplasty because obviously of chronic rejection the cartilage in the transplanted knee joint vanished. One patient received this additional total knee arthroplasty fifteen months following transplantation, one patient 35 months post-transplant and one patient 50 months post-transplant. Two years after transplantation possibly due to a lack of proprioception in his allograft, one patient developed a fatigue fracture of the tibial head of his transplanted knee joint while running downstairs. Also in this case we decided to perform an additional total knee arthroplasty using part of the remaining transplanted joint bone as a base. Post-operatively this patient was pain-free with a stable joint, good mobility and the ability to walk and returned to work. Unfortunately this patient developed a deep infection in the operated knee joint two years later. At that time due to social and private reasons this patient decided not to continue limb saving procedures. He preferred to bring his hospital career to a definitive end by a thigh amputation.

Discussion

The first vascularized allogeneic transplantations of bone and total knee joints introduced a supplementary option to orthopedic surgery. Both procedures offer a last line of defence to patients whose only other alternative would be a fused knee joint or an amputation. It is not and never was intended to replace established treatments. From the technically point of view the vascularized transplantation of femoral diaphysis and knee joint allografts seems to be possible. As far as biomechanical properties and the facilitation of revascularization are concerned intramedullary nailing for osteosynthesis between recipient and donor bone seem to provide superior results compared to other osteosynthesis. Cyclosporine A and azathioprine immunosuppression do not appear to have an adverse effect on bone healing and osseous consolidation of osteotomies.

Human bone has proved to be an immunological target even in non-vascularized bone transplantation [9, 10]. Therefore immunosuppressive treatment is essential to protect allogeneic vessels, bone, cartilage, synovial and tendon tissues from rejection. But obviously cyclosporine A and azathioprine immunosuppression in the doses we used were not effective in completely suppressing acute and chronic rejection episodes. While in all three cases of femoral diaphysis transplants it was not necessary to continue drug immunosuppression beyond the time of osseous incorporation of the grafts it seems to be unavoidable to continue immunosuppression following transplantation of the novel joints life long. Another unresolved problem that must be addressed is the accurate monitoring of rejection episodes in the bone allografts. Vascularized bone allografts are slow-flow organs. This in combination with the antigenicity of the accompanying vascular tissues may pose and increase the risk of graft thrombosis leading to necrosis. Whether or not anticoagulation is mandatory and for how long is open for discussion. Finally, we would like to mention the problem that the knee joint transplants get denervated during harvest. This could potentially lead to a neuropathic arthropathy. Propioception of the joint allograft appears to be absent due to bone and joint denervation. This could lead to repeated unperceived microtraumatisation and also fractures of the transplant as a consequence.

However further investigations are necessary until vascularized bone and joint transplantation will have the potential to become established alternatives in orthopedic surgery.

References

1. Chiron P, Colombier JA, Tricoire JL, Puget J, Utheza G, Glodl Y, Puel P. Une allogreffe massive vascularisée de diaphyse fémorale chez l'homme. *Int Orthop* 1990; 14: 269-72.
2. Clohisy DR, Mankin HJ. Osteoarticular allografts for reconstruction after resection of a musculoskeletal tumor in the proximal end of the tibia. *J Bone Jt Surg* 1994; 76A: 549-54.
3. Doi K, Akino T, Shigetomi M, Maramatsu K, Kawai S. Vascularized bone allografts: review of current concept. *Microsurgery* 1994; 15: 831-41.
4. Hofmann GO, Kirschner MH, Bühren V, Land W. Allogeneic vascularized transplantation of a human femoral diaphysis under cyclosporine A immunosuppression. *Transplant Int* 1995; 8: 418-9.
5. Hofmann GO, Kirschner MH, Wagner FD, Land W, Bühren V. First vascularized knee joint transplantation in man. *Tx Med* 1996; 8: 46-7.

6. Hofmann GO, Kirschner MH, Wagner FD, Land W, Bühren V. Allogeneic vascularized grafting of a human knee joint with postoperative immunosuppression. *Arch Orthop Trauma Surg* 1997; 116: 125-8.
7. Hofmann GO, Kirschner MH. Clinical experience in allogeneic vascularized bone and joint allografting. *Microsurgery* 2000; 20: 375-83.
8. Kirschner MH, Wagner FD, Nerlich A, Land W, Bühren V, Hofmann GO. Allogeneic grafting of vascularized bone segments under immunosupression clinical results of the transplantation of femoral diaphysis. *Transpl Int* 1998; 11: 195-203.
9. Hofmann GO, Falk C, Wangemann T. Immunological transformations in the recipient's of grafted allogeneic human bone. *Arch Orthop Trauma Surg* 1997; 116: 143-50.
10. Ortiz-Cruz E, Gebhardt MC, Jennings LC, Springfield DS, Mankin HJ. The results of transplantation of intercalary allografts after resection of tumors. *J Bone Jt Surg* 1997; 79 A: 97-106.

Composite Tissue Allografts
Dubernard J.-M., ed.
© John Libbey Eurotext, Paris, 2001

Allogeneic hematopoietic stem cell transplantation: current issues and future prospects

Gérard Socié, Eliane Gluckman
Service de Greffe de Moelle, Hôpital Saint-Louis, Paris, France

Major developments have occurred in the field of hematopoietic stem cell transplantation since the first successful transplants from HLA-identical siblings in the late 60's. The formally experimental procedure has become established therapy for a number of congenital or acquired disorders of the hematopoietic system and for chemotherapy-sensitive malignancies. Reduced transplant-related mortality has led to a widening of indications. The rapid increase in utilization of this technique over the past few years has been documented by the surveys of the International Bone Marrow Transplant Registry (IBMTR) [1] and annual transplant activity report of the European Group for Blood and Marrow Transplantation (EBMT) [2]. Traditional bone marrow transplantation has been supplemented by transplantation of hematopoietic stem and progenitor cells from different stem cell sources and donor types. Blood and marrow transplantation today includes allogeneic transplants from bone marrow, peripheral blood, cord blood, as a stem cell source. Donors for allogeneic transplants can be HLA-identical siblings, HLA-mismatched relatives or unrelated volunteers. Here, we summarize some current issues and future prospects in allogeneic stem cell transplantation. We do not attempt to be exhaustive, readers with interest in the field will find much more details in two reference text books [3, 4].

Stem cell sources

Peripheral blood stem cell transplantation

Traditionally, hematopoietic stem cells for transplantation were obtained from bone marrow. In the 1980s it was shown that autologous cells harvested from blood could restore hematopoiesis, that large numbers of these cells could be obtained after administration of hematopoietic growth factors, and that blood derived cells provided more rapid hematopoietic recovery than bone marrow (review in [5]). More than 90% of autotransplants done in Europe in 1996 were performed using peripheral blood stem cells [2]. In 1995, three centers reported rapid hematopoietic recovery and acceptable acute graft-*versus*-host disease (GvHD) after such allografts from HLA-identical relatives [6-8]. About 2,500 blood allografts were reported to the IBMTR between 1994 and 1997 and 20% of the number of allografts reported to the EBMT in 1996 [1, 2]. However, some single center studies pointed out that such transplants might be associated with an increased risk of chronic GvHD, especially in older patients [9, 10].

Whether or not, peripheral blood stem cell can safely replace bone marrow in allogeneic stem cell transplantation was thus an open question. Two randomized studies have recently explored this issue. In a single center American study, 172 patients with hematological cancer were randomly assigned to receive either bone marrow or mobilized peripheral-blood cells from HLA-identical relatives [11]. The recovery of both neutrophils and platelets was faster with peripheral-blood cells than with marrow. The cumulative incidence of grade II, III, or IV acute GvHD was 64 percent with peripheral-blood cells and 57 percent with marrow (hazard ratio, 1.21, $p = 0.35$). The cumulative incidence of chronic GvHD was 46 percent with peripheral-blood cells and 35 percent with marrow (hazard ratio, 1.16, $p = 0.54$). The estimated overall probability of survival at two years was 66 percent with peripheral-blood cells and 54 percent with marrow (hazard ratio for death, 0.62, $p = 0.06$).The rate of disease-free survival at two years was 65 percent with peripheral-blood cells and 45 percent with marrow (hazard ratio for relapse or death, 0.60; $p = 0.03$). In a French multicenter trial, 111 patients with leukemia in the early stages and with HLA-matched sibling donors were randomized [12]. One hundred one underwent transplantation. Patients in the peripheral blood cell group reached suitable platelet and neutrophil level earlier than did the BMT group. However, patients who received a peripheral blood cell graft had significantly more chronic GvHD but survival rates were similar. Thus, today we still need more prolonged follow-up to know if peripheral blood can safely replace marrow cells in allogeneic stem cell transplantation.

Umbilical cord blood transplantation

Since the first cord blood transplant (CBT) performed in 1988 [13], cord blood transplantation is increasingly used as a new source of hematopoietic stem cells. In order to analyze factors associated with outcome of cord blood transplants, Eurocord-Cord Blood Transplant Group collected data on CBT provided by more than 80 centers in 20 countries. The analysis of clinical results has shown that related cord blood transplants give better outcome than unrelated cord blood transplants in some but not all indications. Factors associated with better survival in related and unrelated cord blood transplants were younger age, and diagnosis with better results in inborn errors and in children with acute leukemia in 1st or 2nd remission. Higher number of nucleated cells in the graft and recipient negative CMV serology were also favorable factors for survival [14].

With the increased number of cord blood transplants analyzed, it is time to try to answer the questions which will help making the choice of the source of stem cells in various clinical situations.

The first question about the general use of cord blood for allogeneic hematopoietic stem cell transplantation has been the concern about the engraftment potential of a single cord blood unit in patients with all hematological conditions and all weights. We and others have shown that a high number of nucleated cells infused is a good prognostic factor for engraftment and survival. For example, in unrelated CBT, patients who received less than 3.7×10^7 nucleated cells/kg had a median time to reach $\geq 500\mu l$ neutrophil of 34 days (range 14 to 48 days) and a median time to reach $\geq 20,000/\mu l$ platelets of 134 days (range 30 to 180 days), while in patients who received more than the median cell dose, the median times were respectively 25 days (range 10 to 56 days) for ANC and 47 days (range 9 to 85 days) for platelets recovery. In order to improve the speed of engraftment, several methods can be investigated as the use of hematopoietic growth factors such as G-CSF, kit ligand or thrombopoietin (TPO). At this stage, the usefulness of these factors has not been demonstrated and deserves further investigation. Another approach could be to expand *in vitro* cord blood progenitors to improve short-term engraftment. This area of investigation seems particularly interesting, as *in vitro* studies have shown that expansion was increased in cord blood compared to bone marrow cells.

Another question is whether GvHD is reduced after cord blood transplantation. One of the first concern raised by the use of cord blood for allogeneic transplant was the possibility of inadvertent transplant of cells of maternal origin. We [15], and other authors, have shown that, indeed, maternal cells were always present in cord blood but that their number was insufficient to induce GvHD. Immunological immaturity of cord blood cells might decrease the incidence and severity of acute GvHD even in HLA mismatched situation. In a joined Eurocord IBMTR study, data on 113 recipients of cord blood from HLA-identical siblings were compared with those of 2,052 recipients of bone marrow from HLA-identical siblings [16]. The study population consisted of children 15 years age or younger. Multivariate analysis demonstrated a lower risk of acute GvHD (relative risk, 0.41; $p = 0.001$) and chronic GvHD (relative risk, 0.35; $p = 0.02$) among recipients of cord-blood. Mortality was similar in the two groups (relative risk of death in the recipients of cord blood, 1.15; $p = 0.43$). Thus recipients of cord-blood transplants from HLA-identical siblings have a lower incidence of acute and chronic GvHD than recipients of bone marrow transplants from HLA-identical siblings.

Finally, one could ask what is the place of cord blood transplant compared to other sources of hematopoietic stem cells. In a recent Eurocord study, in order to compare the outcomes of unrelated umbilical cord blood transplants (UCBTs) or bone marrow transplants [17], 541 children with acute leukemia (AL) transplanted with umbilical cord blood (n = 99), T-cell-depleted unrelated bone marrow transplants (T-UBMT) (n = 180), or non-manipulated (UBMT) (n = 262), were analyzed in a retrospective multicenter study. The major difference between the 3 groups was the higher number in the UCBT group of HLA mismatches. After adjustment, differences in outcomes appeared in the first 100 days after the transplantation. Compared with UBMT recipients, UCBT recipients had delayed hematopoietic recovery (Hazard ratio [HR] = 0.37), increased 100 day transplant-related mortality (HR = 2.13) and decreased acute GvHD (HR = 0.50). T-UBMT recipients had decreased acute GvHD (HR = 0.25) and increased risk of relapse (HR 5 1). After day 100 post-transplant, the 3 groups achieved similar results in terms of relapse. Chronic GvHD was decreased after T-UBMT (HR = 0.21) and UCBT (HR = 0.24), and overall mortality was higher in T-UBMT recipients (HR =). In conclusion, the use of UCBT, as a source of hematopoietic stem cells, is a reasonable option for children with AL lacking an acceptably matched unrelated marrow donor.

At this stage, we recommend searching simultaneously Bone Marrow Donor Registries and Cord Blood Banks. The final decision must take into account the degree of HLA identity, the availability of the donor, the speed of search, the urgency of the transplant, the number of cells present in the cord blood and in the case of unrelated bone marrow donor transplants, the donor age, sex, number of pregnancies and CMV status.

Allogeneic stem cell transplantation from donors other than HLA-identical siblings

Allogeneic stem cell transplantation from unrelated volunteers

Only 25-30% of patients have an HLA-matched sibling donor. To overcome this problem, potential bone marrow donors, now numbering over 5 million, were recruited by over 50 registries worldwide. In 1997, more than 3,500 transplantations were performed with use of marrow from such donors. Because of the extreme polymorphism of the HLA system, only about 60% of patients without a family donor find an unrelated donor. Large series of patients who underwent transplantation from an unrelated donor are now available. The main problem in the interpretation of the results comes from the definition of an "HLA-matched" unrelated donors. First transplants were performed using the definition of a "matched" using serology. We now know that the multigene HLA-family has at least 12 polymorphic loci. As a results first transplants were associated with high incidences of severe acute GvHD and rejection of the graft [18-20]. The advent of molecular typing of HLA-class II molecule lead to the recognition of the role of DRB1 and DQB1 HLA mismatching in the genesis of acute GvHD and more recently of HLA-C in graft rejection [21-23]. With the use of unrelated donors matched at the HLA-A and B loci serologically and at the DRB1 locus by molecular biology, the Seattle group recently reported long-term survival rates above 50% in patient grafted for chronic myelogenous leukemia [24]. The 5-year survival rate was even more impressive (74%) in those patients who were less than 50 years of age and who were transplanted within one year of diagnosis. Another single center study also reported recently a similar outcome of transplantation with matched sibling or unrelated-donor bone marrow in children with leukemia [25]. Although encouraging, these results should however be interpreted with caution since unrelated transplants are still currently associated with a higher transplant-related mortality as compared with matched sibling transplants [26]. Current issue in unrelated transplants is to explore the effect of molecular matching of class I alleles. Two recent studies suggest that genomic typing of class I HLA alleles adds substantially to the success of such transplants [27, 28]. Future prospects will include the role (if any) of T-cell depletion of the graft and if "permissive" mismatches do exist.

Allogeneic stem cell transplantation from mismatched related donors

While transplantation from a 1-locus mismatched related donor seems to lead to similar outcome than matched sibling transplants [26], this is a relatively rare situation. More recently some groups re-explored the role of haplo-identical related donors (*i.e.* 3 antigen mismatched), a far more common genetic situation (mother, father, sibling...). Although feasible now using high dose peripheral stem-cell and T-cell depletion, these transplants are associated with a profound and long-lasting immune deficiency, and should thus be considered as experimental [29-32].

Hematopoietic stem cell plasticity

Stem cells have traditionally been characterized as either embryonic (pluripotent) or organ-specific. Recent work suggests that latter can "transdifferentiate" into other cell types, carrying significant implications for possible clinical use of these cells.

Recently, stem cells have been prospectively isolated using combinations of surface markers. Such prospective isolation has been achieved for blood-forming HSC, peripheral nervous system (PNS) stem cells and central nervous system (CNS) stem cells. CNS stem cells have also been isolated by selective growth in cultures. Stem cells have been enriched, but perhaps not yet isolated, from a number of rapidly regenerating tissues such as skin, intestine, skeletal muscle and a variety of mesenchymal derivatives. Although several papers claim new stem-cell discoveries or transplantation, the stem-cell appellation is only deserved in those studies that identify and/or transplant isolated, clonogenic, self-renewing and differentiating progenitor cells [33].

A long-standing concept has been that organ-specific stem cells are restricted to making the differentiated cell types of the tissue in which they reside. In other words, they have irreversibly lost the capacity to generate other cell types in the body. This character of restriction fundamentally distinguishes organ-specific stem cells from ES cells. The concept of developmental restriction has received considerable support from classical embryological experiments showing that pieces of undifferentiated tissue transplanted from one region of the embryo to another rapidly lose the ability to be respecified by their novel host environment.

A recent series of studies, however, has challenged the notion of lineage-restriction in organ-specific stem cells. These experiments have been interpreted as evidence that adult stem cells from one tissue or organ can be induced to differentiate into cells of other organs, either *in vitro* or after transplantation *in vivo*. One of the first provocative demonstrations was bone-marrow-derived cells that were found to target and differentiate into muscle [34]. Then there came reports that adult neural-cell cultures containing neural stem cells could differentiate into blood cells [35]. A flurry of studies followed that reported bone-marrow-to-brain, bone-marrow-derived stroma-to-brain, bone-marrow-to-liver, skin-to-brain, brain-to-heart and other such stem cell differentiation [36]. If correct, the findings would imply that either organ-specific stem cells can overcome their intrinsic restrictions upon exposure to a novel environment ("transdifferentiate"), perhaps *via* genomic reprogramming, or alternatively, the concept of developmental restriction in organ-specific stem cells is wrong. In the latter case, there would be essentially no intrinsic difference between organ-specific stem cells and ES cells. These results also have potentially important practical as well as theoretical implications: for example, the difficulty in expanding certain kinds of stem cells (for example, HSC) *ex vivo* to increase their number could be overcome by substituting stem cells from other tissues that are easier to grow, such as neural stem cells; conversely, stem cells that are difficult to access for autologous grafting, such as neural stem cells, could be substituted by stem cells that are more easily accessible, such as HSC.

References

1. Horowitz MM, Rowlings PA. An update from the International Bone Marrow Transplant Registry and the Autologous Blood and Marrow Transplant Registry on current activity in hematopoietic stem cell transplantation. *Curr Opin Hematol* 1997; 4: 395-400.
2. Gratwohl A, Passweg J, Baldomero H, Hermans J. Blood and marrow transplantation activity in Europe 1996. *Bone Marrow Transplant* 1998; 22: 227-40.
3. Forman SJ, Blume KG, Thomas ED. *Bone marrow transplantation*, 2nd ed. Cambridge, Ma: Blackwell Scientific, 1998.
4. Barrett J, Treleaven J. *The clinical practice of stem-cell transplantation*. Oxford: Isis Medical Media Ltd, 1998.
5. Armitage JO. Bone marrow transplantation. *N Engl J Med* 1994; 330: 827-38.
6. Bensinger WI, Weaver CH, Appelbaum FR, Rowley S, Demirer T, Sanders J, et al. Transplantation of allogeneic peripheral blood stem cells mobilized by recombinant human granulocyte colony-stimulating factor. *Blood* 1995; 85: 1655-8.
7. Korbling M, Przepiorka D, Huh YO, Engel H, Vanbesien K, Giralt S, et al. Allogeneic blood stem cell transplantation for refractory leukemia and lymphoma: Potential advantage of blood over marrow allografts. *Blood* 1995; 85: 1659-65.
8. Schmitz N, Dreger P, Suttorp M, Rohwedder EB, Haferlach T, Loffler H, et al. Primary transplantation of allogeneic peripheral blood progenitor cells mobilized by filgrastim (granulocyte colony – stimulating factor). *Blood* 1995; 85: 1666-72.
9. Bensinger WI, Clift RA, Anasetti C, Appelbaum FA, Demirer T, Rowley S, et al. Transplantation of allogeneic peripheral blood stem cells mobilized by recombinant human granulocyte colony stimulating factor. *Stem Cells* 1996; 14: 90-105.
10. Bacigalupo A, Zikos P, Vanlint MT, Valbonesi M, Lamparelli T, Gualandi F, et al. Allogeneic bone marrow or peripheral blood cell transplants in adults with hematologic malignancies: A single-center experience. *Exp Hematol* 1998; 26: 409-14.
11. Bensinger WI, Martin PJ, Storer B, Clift R, Forman SJ, Negrin R, et al. Transplantation of bone marrow as compared with peripheral-blood cells from HLA-identical relatives in patients with hematologic cancers. *N Engl J Med* 2001; 344: 175-81.
12. Blaise D, Kuentz M, Fortanier C, Bourhis JH, Milpied N, Sutton L, et al. Randomized trial of bone marrow *versus* lenograstim-primed blood cell allogeneic transplantation in patients with early-stage leukemia: A report from the Societe Francaise de Greffe de Moelle. *J Clin Oncol* 2000; 18: 537-46.
13. Gluckman E, Broxmeyer HE, Auerbach AD, Friedman H, Douglas GW, Devergie A, et al. Hematopoietic reconstitution in a patient with Fanconi anemia by means of umbilical-cord blood from an HLA-identical sibling. *N Engl J Med* 1989; 321: 1174-8.
14. Gluckman E, Rocha V, Boyerchammard A, Locatelli F, Arcese W, Pasquini R, et al. Outcome of cord-blood transplantation from related and unrelated donors. *N Engl J Med* 1997; 337: 373-81.
15. Petit T, Gluckman E, Carosella E, Brossard Y, Brison O, Socie G. A highly sensitive polymerase chain reaction method reveals the ubiquitous presence of maternal cells in human umbilical cord blood. *Exp Hematol* 1995; 23: 1601-5.
16. Rocha V, Wagner JE, Sobocinski KA, Klein JP, Zhang MJ, Horowitz MM, et al. Graft-*versus*-host disease in children who have received a cord-blood or bone marrow transplant from an HLA-Identical sibling. *N Engl J Med* 2000; 342: 1846-54.
17. Rocha V, Cornish J, Sievers EL, Filipovich A, Locatelli F, Peters C, et al. Comparison of outcomes of unrelated bone marrow and umbilical cord blood transplants in children with acute leukemia. *Blood* 2001; 97: 2962-71.
18. Devergie A, Apperley JF, Labopin M, Madrigal A, Jacobsen N, Carreras E, et al. European results of matched unrelated donor bone marrow transplantation for chronic myeloid leukemia. Impact of HLA class II matching. *Bone Marrow Transplant* 1997; 20: 11-9.

19. Mcglave P, Bartsch G, Anasetti C, Ash R, Beatty P, Gajewski J, et al. Unrelated Donor Marrow Transplantation Therapy for Chronic Myelogenous Leukemia – Initial Experience of the National Marrow Donor Program. *Blood* 1993; 81: 543-50.
20. Kernan NA, Bartsch G, Ash RC, Beatty PG, Champlin R, Filipovich A, et al. Analysis of 462 Transplantations from Unrelated Donors Facilitated by the National Marrow Donor Program. *N Engl J Med* 1993; 328: 593-602.
21. Petersdorf EW, Longton GM, Anasetti C, Martin PJ, Mickelson EM, Smith AG, et al. The significance of HLA-DRB1 matching on clinical outcome after HLA-A, B, DR identical unrelated donor marrow transplantation. *Blood* 1995; 86: 1606-13.
22. Petersdorf EW, Longton GM, Anasetti C, Mickelson EM, Mckinney SK, Smith AG, et al. Association of HLA-C disparity with graft failure after marrow transplantation from unrelated donors. *Blood* 1997; 89: 1818-23.
23. Petersdorf EW, Longton GM, Anasetti C, Mickelson EM, Smith AG, Martin PJ, et al. Definition of HLA-DQ as a transplantation antigen. *Proc Natl Acad Sci USA* 1996; 93: 15358-63.
24. Hansen JA, Gooley TA, Martin PJ, Appelbaum F, Chauncey TR, Clift RA, et al. Bone marrow transplants from unrelated donors for patients with chronic myeloid leukemia. *N Engl J Med* 1998; 338: 962-8.
25. Hongeng S, Krance RA, Bowman LC, Srivastava DK, Cunningham JM, Horwitz EM, et al. Outcomes of transplantation with matched – sibling and unrelated – donor bone marrow in children with leukaemia. *Lancet* 1997; 350: 767-71.
26. Szydlo R, Goldman JM, Klein JP, Gale RP, Ash RC, Bach FH, et al. Results of allogeneic bone marrow transplants for leukemia using donors other than HLA-identical siblings. *J Clin Oncol* 1997; 15: 1767-77.
27. Sasazuki T, Juji T, Morishima Y, Kinukawa N, Kashiwabara H, Inoko H, et al. Effect of matching of class I HLA alleles on clinical outcome after transplantation of hematopoietic stem cells from an unrelated donor. *N Engl J Med* 1998; 339: 1177-85.
28. Petersdorf EW, Gooley TA, Anasetti C, Martin PJ, Smith AG, Mickelson EM, et al. Optimizing outcome after unrelated marrow transplantation by comprehensive matching of HLA class I and II alleles in the donor and recipient. *Blood* 1998; 92: 3515-20.
29. Aversa F, Tabilio A, Terenzi A, Velardi A, Falzetti F, Giannoni C, et al. Successful engraftment of T-cell-depleted haploidentical "three- loci" incompatible transplants in leukemia patients by addition of recombinant human granulocyte colony – stimulating factor – mobilized peripheral blood progenitor cells to bone marrow inoculum. *Blood* 1994; 84: 3948-55.
30. Henslee Downey PJ, Abhyankar SH, Parrish RS, Pati AR, Godder KT, Neglia WJ, et al. Use of partially mismatched related donors extends access to allogeneic marrow transplant. *Blood* 1997; 89: 3864-72.
31. Aversa F, Tabilio A, Velardi A, Cunningham I, Terenzi A, Falzetti F, et al. Treatment of high-risk acute luekemia with T-cell depleted stem cells from related donors with one fully mismatched HLA haplotype. *N Engl J Med* 1998; 339: 1186-93.
32. Aversa F, Martelli MF, Reisner Y. Hematopoietic stem-cell transplantation for acute leukemia. *N Engl J Med* 1999; 340: 811-2.
33. Anderson DJ, Gage FH, Weissman IL. Can stem cells cross lineage boundaries? *Nat Med* 2001; 7: 393-5.
34. Ferrari G, Cusella-De Angelis G, Coletta M, Paolucci E, Stornaiuolo A, Cossu G, et al. Muscle regeneration by bone marrow-derived myogenic progenitors. *Science* 1998; 279: 1528-30.
35. Bjornson CRR, Rietze RL, Reynolds BA, Magli MC, Vescovi AL. Turning brain into blood: A hematopoietic fate adopted by adult neural stem cells in vivo. *Science* 1999; 283: 534-7.
36. Morrison SJ. Stem cell potential: can anything make anything? *Curr Biol* 2001; 11: R7-R9.

Pathology of the skin after hand allografting

Jean Kanitakis, Denis Jullien
Department of Dermatology, Ed. Herriot Hospital, Lyon, France

In September 1998 and Junuary 2000 the first simple and double human hand allografts were performed in Lyon by an international team headed by Pr J.-M. Dubernard. The recipients, a 48- (R1) and a 36-year-old (R2) white man received their allografts from brain-dead donors with whom they shared the same blood group but not all HLA alleles. Details concerning the surgical procedure and immunosuppressive treatment have previously been reported [1-4]. The aim of the present study was to monitor a potential rejection of the allografted limb, and to assess the quality of the allografted skin. The patients underwent regularly clinical examination of the skin of the allografted hand. Sequential skin biopsies were taken from the grafted forearms from day 5 up to month 28 post-graft (when the allograft of R1 was removed due to non-compliance of the immunosuppressive treatment resulting in chronic graft rejection), and from day 0 to month 18 post-graft (R2). Frozen and paraffin-embedded tissue sections were examined by conventional histology and immunohistochemistry, using a wide panel of antibodies recognizing various skin cell types.

Around the 7th-8th week post-graft, both recipients presented well-demarcated, occasionally confluent erythematous, slightly infiltrated macules over the allografted skin of the forearm. Histologically these comprised a dense dermal, mainly perivascular mononuclear cell infiltrate; it consisted predominantly of $CD3^+CD4^+$ lymphocytes, with occasional $CD8^+$ lymphocytes and histiocyte-like cells of recipient's origin, as shown by the expression of the recipient's specific HLA-A24 antigen. These findings were considered as signs of acute (cutaneous) graft rejection, and were reversed with an increase of the immunosuppressive treatment and addition of local steroids and tacrolimus ointment [5].

During the 14th month, R1 presented red-violaceous, scaly, slightly infiltrated lesions mainly on the dorsum of the hand and the periungueal areas of the allografted limb; histologically these showed epidermal thickening (hypergranulosis, acanthosis, papillomatosis), vacuolar changes of the basal epidermal layer and a band-like subepidermal infiltrate made of $CD3^+$, $CD4^+$ or $CD8^+$ lymphocytes (interface dermatitis). These changes were identical to chronic lichenoid GvHD, and were considered as chronic (cutaneous) graft rejection [6]; they improved slightly under local steroid treatment but progressively worsened because of non-compliance with the immunosuppressive treatment, and resulted in diffuse, erythematous-scaly, psoriasiform lesions involving the majority of the skin of the allograft.

This was removed 28 months after grafting, and examined histologically. The major changes were seen in the skin, that showed the same changes as those seen earlier, albeit to a more severe degree, including now areas of epidermal necrosis. Remarkably, the underlying tissues (tendons, bone and muscles) did not show major changes, except from a mild perivascular infiltrate found within the muscular tissue.

Aside from these acute and chronic graft rejection episodes, the skin showed histologically a normal appearance, including the epidermis, epidermal adnexae (hair follicles and eccrine sweat glands), blood vessels, nerves and adipose tissue. Immunohistologically, most cell types of the skin were present immediately post-graft and remained detectable throughout the study period. These included cycling ($Ki67^+$) epidermal and adnexal keratinocytes, $CD1a^+/S100^+/Lag^+/Langerin^+$ epidermal Langerhans cells (LC), $S100^+/MART-1^+$ melanocytes, factor $XIIIa^+$ and $CD34^+$ dermal dendrocytes, $CD34^+$/von Willebrand factor$^+$ endothelial cells, $S100^+$ Schwann cells, epithelial membrane antigen$^+$ perineural fibroblasts and desmin$^+$ smooth muscle cells. Epidermal keratinocytes expressed normally keratin immunoreactivity. The density of LC was normal, and from day 77 post-graft the epidermis of the allograft (R1) harbored some LC of recipient's origin (microchimerism), recognized thanks to the double expression of the CD1a and the HLA-A24 antigens [5]. Epidermal Merkel cells (keratin 20^+) were first detected during the 12th month. Axons remained undetectable until the 6th (R2) or the 15th months (R1), when neurofilament immunoreactivity was observed within dermal nerves. The quantity of dermal axons increased regularly within the following weeks, and free (unmyelinated) nerve endings were also observed in the papillary dermis (R1). Remarkably, this restoration of cutaneous innervation paralleled the recovery of superficial skin sensitivity [7]. Nerve fibers were detected within the epidermis and arrector pili muscles thanks to immunoreactivity for PGP9.5 and neuron-specific enolase respectively, during the 15th month (R2).

Our results show that in this composite tissue allograft, the skin is a privileged target of graft rejection. Clinical and pathological monitoring of this tissue is a reliable test to detect early an acute and chronic rejection in the setting of human hand allografts (and likely also after allografting of other composite tissues). Aside from rejection episodes, the allografted skin maintains a normal structure and trophicity. Cells present within the allograft (such as epidermal keratinocytes and endothelial cells) remain viable. Cells from recipient's origin (such as LC and dermal axons) progressively colonize the graft, resulting in a microchimerism that may facilitate graft tolerance [8].

References

1. Dubernard JM, Owen E, Herzberg G, Lanzetta M, Martin X, Kapila H, Dawahra M, Hakim N. Human hand allograft: report on first 6 months. *Lancet* 1999; 353: 1315-20.
2. Dubernard JM, Owen E, Lefrançois N, Petruzzo P, Martin X, Dawahra M, Jullien D, Kanitakis J, Francès C, Preville X, Gebuhrer L, Hakim N, Lanzetta M, Kapila H, Herzberg G, Revillard JP. First human hand transplantation. *Transpl Int* 2000; 13 (Suppl. 1): S521-4.
3. Petruzzo P, Lefrançois N, Kanitakis J, Gebuhrer L, Da Silva M, Konan PG, Dawahra M, Martin X, Revillard JP, Dubernard JM. Immunosuppression in composite tissue allograft. *Transpl Proc* 2001; 33: 2398-9.

4. Petruzzo P, Revillard JP, Kanitakis J, Lanzetta M, Herzberg G, Lefrançois N, Owen M, Dubernard JM. First double hand transplantation: efficacy, risks and functional results achieved with a conventional immunosuppressive protocol (submitted).
5. Kanitakis J, Jullien D, Nicolas JF, Francès C, Claudy A, Revillard JP, Owen M, Dubernard JM. Sequential histological and immunohistochemical study of the skin of the first human hand allograft. *Transplantation* 2000; 69: 1380-5.
6. Kanitakis J, Jullien D, Francès C, Claudy A, Revillard JP, Owen M, Dubernard JM. Immunohistological studies of the skin of human hand allografts. Our experience with two patients. *Transplant Proc* 2001; 33: 1722.
7. Kanitakis J, Jullien D, De Boer B, Claudy A, Dubernard JM. Regeneration of cutaneous innervation in the first human hand allograft. *Lancet* 2000; 356: 1738-9.
8. Kanitakis J, Jullien D, Claudy A, Revillard JP, Dubernard JM. Microchimerism in a human hand allograft. *Lancet* 1999; 354: 1820-1.

Human Hand Allografts

Hand transplantation: Lyon experience

Palmina Petruzzo, Jean-Michel Dubernard
Service de Chirurgie de la Transplantation, Hôpital Édouard-Herriot, Lyon, France

A composite tissue allograft (CTA) such as hand transplantation is an ideal replacement for missing tissue after traumatic loss, tumor resection or congenital absence by supplying near-identical part by a cadaveric donor for reconstruction. The success of any composite tissue allograft depends on prevention of host rejection and his functional recovery. The introduction of new immunosuppressant agents like FK506 and mycophenolate mofetil, especially in combination, resulted in long-term CTA viability in large animal models [1, 2]. Improvement in detection of rejection and experience in the treatment of this event increased the degree of success in viability and function of the transplanted limbs [2].

Despite the limitations inherent in animal models, functional recovery of CTA with adequate immunosuppression appeared to be comparable to that occurred in upper extremity replantation, with the advantage that hand transplantation can be planned and executed electively.

Based on these findings we performed the first human hand allotransplantation in September 1998 [3, 4], followed by several cases in USA, China, Italy [5, 6] and by the first double hand transplantation performed in Lyon in January 2000, followed by other cases in Austria and China.

Material and methods

In the first case, performed on 23rd September 1998, the recipient was a 48 years old man who suffered a traumatic amputation of his right forearm in 1984. After a replantation, he was reamputated in 1989 because of function lack. In the second case, performed on 13th January 2000, the recipient was a 33 years old man who suffered a traumatic amputation of both hands in 1996. Myoelectric protheses were employed after the accident. In both cases T and B cell cross match was negative.

The recipients underwent routine pre-transplantation investigations and specific morphological and functional tests of forearm stumps such as arteriography, muscle and nerve charts, electromyography and functional magnetic resonance imaging.

In both cases patients were intensively informed and consulted as well as psychologically assessed by a psychiatric team to be sure of patient's ability to cope with the transplantation.

In both cases donor brachial artery was dissected and cannulated, then the limb irrigated with University of Wisconsin solution at 4 °C. Graft anatomical structures were dissected and tagged. Recipients' stumps were prepared: all available muscles and neurovascular structures were dissected and identified. Replantation consisted of sequential bone fixation, arterial and venous anastomosis, nerve sutures, muscle and tendon connection, cutaneous sutures.

Immunosuppressive protocol included an initial induction phase with polyclonal antibodies (thymoglobulin 1.25 mg/kg/d for ten days), tacrolimus (0.2 mg/kg/d with blood levels between 15 and 20 µg/ml in the first month), prednisolone (250 mg on day 1; 1 mg/kg/d for ten days, then slowly tapered to 20 mg/d), mycophenolate mofetil (2 g/d). Monoclonal anti-CD25 antibodies (Simulect) were also used in both patients as the rapid decrease of antithymocyte globulins. The maintenance phase consisted of prednisone (10 mg/d)), tacrolimus (blood trough levels between 5 and 10 µg/ml), mycophenolate mofetil (2,000 mg/d).

Rehabilitation program included physiotherapy, electrostimulation and occupational therapy; it focused on sensory, visual, motor and haptic stimulation of the grafted hands. It started twelve hours after surgery and was performed twice daily for the entire follow-up period.

Follow-up protocol included clinical course, X-rays, bone scintigraphy, arteriography, skin biopsies, electromiography, muscle and nerve charts, functional magnetic resonance (fMRI) and evaluation of sensory and motional recovery. Follow-up period was 29 months for the right hand transplantation and 18 months for the double hand transplantation.

Results

In both recipients skin and wound healing proceeded normally. Allograft skin looked normal with respect to color and temperature as well as hair and nail growth. Histologically the skin showed an overall normal structure.

From day 77 post-transplantation, dendritic cells expressing the recipient HLA-24 antigen were shown in the epidermidis of the first recipient.

Nerve regeneration and functional recovery

In both patients nerve regeneration was demonstrated by skin biopsies, electromyography and sensorimotor tests. Dermal axons detected thanks to neurofilament immunoreactivity were first demonstrated on day 524 and on day 185 post-transplant respectively in right hand and in double hand transplantation. Nerve regeneration was parallel to sensitivity and motility recovery.

In the right hand grafted patient by 3 months Tinel's sign had advanced to 21 cm on the median nerve and 20 cm on the ulnar nerve. At 18 months after transplantation sensitivity studies, such as Semmes Weinstein test, Weber-Moberg test and Dellon test, showed complete recovery of sensitivity to pain, cold and heat in all digits; recovery of vibratory sensitivity in all digits with errors in localization between second and third finger; partial recovery of monofilament sensibility in all fingers but with errors in localization in median nerve territory. No discriminative sensibility in median nerve and in ulnar nerve territory was evidenced. Although he did not improve his motility because of no compliance to the rehabilitation program, at one year he could hold bottles and glasses and write with a pen. At 18 months after transplantation despite the extrinsic musculature was well developed, active range of motion was limited and intrinsic musculature was present in ulnar nerve territory alone, while it was completely absent in median nerve territory.

In the double hand grafted patient by 3 months the presence of Tinel's sign was noted 14 cm from the anastomosis of the left ulnar nerve, 12 cm from the anastomosis left radial nerve and 12 cm from the anastomosis of both right nerves. By six months the sensitivity to needles and thermal stimuli was normal on dorsal and palmar face of both hands and of all fingertips, except the left thumb. By 15 months sensitivity recovery was demonstrated on all fingertips of both hands using 4.56 monofilaments (Semmes-Weinstein test). The patient did not present subjective symptoms such as numbness, paraesthesia and cold intolerance. By 12 months electromyography demonstrated muscle innervation in the ulnar nerve territory and a small innervation in the median nerve territory. At this follow-up point extrinsic musculature was developed well and intrinsic musculature started. By 1 year after transplantation the double hand grafted patient was able to perform the same daily activities that were possible with the myoelectric prostheses, in addition he could perform some activities such as taking care of his personal hygiene, holding a glass, a pen and a phone that were impossible before the transplantation. The patient considered "the" hands as "his own" hands as documented by the psychiatrists. In addition, functional MRI showed that sensorimotor activations, which in pre-transplantation period were found close to the face area, progressively regained the habitual cortical locus (classical hand area) after the transplantation.

Acute and chronic rejection episodes

On day 52 and 77 after transplantation in the first recipient erythematous maculopapules appeared on the dorsal face of the right grafted arm, while on day 57 and 82 in the second recipient maculopapular asymptomatic lesions developed on the left grafted forearm. In both cases skin biopsies revealed a mild dense dermal inflammatory infiltrate predominantly made of lymphocytes of recipient origin. These findings were considered as signs of acute rejection and treated with an increase in oral prednisone and topical application of tacrolimus and clobetasol cream. All the acute rejection episodes resolved clinically and histologically within few days.

At 16 months post-transplant the right hand grafted patient who admitted to take only intermittently the immunosuppressive treatment, presented an episode of skin rejection, which was diagnosed as chronic graft rejection and treated with monoclonal anti-CD25 antibodies and prednisone reintroduction, leading to a slow regression of the lesions. By 24 months post-transplant in the first recipient the complete suspension of immunosuppressive drugs induced a progressive rejection process characterized by edema and necrotic cutaneous lesions. Thus, the patient was amputated 28 months post-transplant. Histologic study of the amputated hand showed lichenoid graft-*versus*-host disease lesions, necrosis of superficial epidermis and epidermal adnexae, a dense cellular infiltrate constituted of recipient lymphocytes in dermis and around dermal vessels. Nerves, muscles, tendons and bones did not show lesions related to the rejection process.

Complications

In the immediate post-operative period anaemia necessitating blood perfusion has been reported in both patients.

On day 8 the second recipient developed antibodies against rabbit globulins with clinical manifestations of serum sickness.

Under the reported immunosuppressive treatment both recipients developed hyperglycemia that was treated with insulin therapy. It disappeared when steroid doses and tacrolimus levels were decreased. In addition, the first recipient presented a temporal increase in creatinine values in correlation with high tacrolimus levels and herpes virus (HSV-1) infection occurred three months post-transplant and it was successfully treated with aciclovir.

No other metabolic or infectious complications related to the immunosuppressive protocol occurred during the follow-up period in the grafted patients.

Discussion

The reconstructive procedure in hand allografts allows to transplant not injured, well-preserved extremities at the most favorable level, without donor-site limitations or morbidity. Consequently, compared with replantation, transplantation of hand allograft can be planned and executed electively with selection of appropriate donors and recipients. The advantages of limb transplantation are contingent upon an effective and safe immunosuppressive protocol. We decided to use the association FK506/MMF/prednisone that is a combination therapy of agents that differ in mechanism of action and in toxicity. American [5] and Italian teams also used this successful immunosuppressive protocol demonstrating that long-term viability in hand allograft is possible with conventional therapeutic levels of immunosuppression.

The acute skin rejection episodes were completely reversed in both recipients increasing steroid oral dose and applying topical immunosuppressant agents. Skin showed to be the principal target of acute and chronic rejection. It is intriguing that in the amputated hand from the first grafted patient the lesions were limited to the skin alone. No chimerism was detected in both patients while Langerhans cells of recipient origin have been demonstrated in the grafted arm of the first transplanted patient [7].

Complete functional restoration is conditioned by nerve regeneration and his event has been demonstrated by the immunohistochemical studies of the skin [8], electromyography and sensitive recovery tests. Nerve regeneration was faster than in the autoreconstructions as FK506 seems to accelerate axonal regeneration [9] increasing the synthesis of axotomy-induced growth-associated protein (GAP-43). Therefore, in the double hand transplantation electromyographic data, passive and active ROM evaluation tests showed a relevant sensorimotor recovery with reinnervation of extrinsic and intrinsic muscles.

Furthermore, fMRI results have demonstrated that peripheral input can modify cortical hand organization in sensorimotor regions demonstrating human brain plasticity [10]. The importance of the rehabilitation program in the future of the upper extremity transplantation has been demonstrated. Our rehabilitation program was complex and intensive including physiotherapy, electro-stimulation and occupational therapy as its final goal was to co-operate to the process of cortical reorganization, which seems to conditionate functional recovery of transplanted hands. Finally but not ultimately, we wish to stress the fact that patient compliance and motivation critically affect the ultimate outcome following hand transplantation.

Acknowledgements

The authors wish to thank for their help the surgical team (X. Martin, M. Dawahra, M. Lanzetta, G. Herzberg, E. Owen, N.S. Hakim), J.P. Revillard, N. Lefrançois, J. Kanitakis, D. Jullien, P. Giraux, A. Sirigu, H. Parmentier, B. Vallet and the team from Val Rosay, the team from La Villa Richelieu.

References

1. Jones JW, Ustuner ET, Zdichavsky M, *et al.* Long-term survival of an extremity composite tissue allograft with FK506-mycophenolate mofetil therapy. *Surgery* 1999; 126: 384-8.
2. Jensen JN, Mackinnon SE. Composite Tissue Allotransplantation: a comprehensive review of the literature-Part II. *J Reconstr Microsurgery* 2000; 16: 235-51.
3. Dubernard JM, Owen E, Herzberg G, Lanzetta M, Martin X, Kapila H, Dawahra M, Hakim NS. Human hand allograft: report on first 6 months. *Lancet* 1999; 353: 1315-20.
4. Dubernard JM, Owen E, Lefrancois N, Petruzzo P, Martin X, Dawahra M, Juillen D, Kanitakis J, Frances C, Preville X, Gebuhrer L, Hakim N, Lanzetta M, Kapila H, Herzberg G, Revillard JP. First human hand transplantation. *Transpl Int* 2000; 13 (Supl.) 19: 521-4.
5. Jones JW, Gruber SA, Barker JH, Breindenbach WC. Successful hand transplantation: one year follow-up. *N Engl J Med* 2000; 343: 468-73.
6. Francois CG, Bredeinbach WC, Maldonado C, Kakoulidis TP, Hodges A, Dubernard JM, Owen E, Pei G, Ren X, Barker JH. Hand transplantation: comparison and observations of the first four clinical cases. *Microsurgery* 2000; 20: 360-71.
7. Kanitakis J, Juillen D, Nicolas JF, Frances C, Claudy A, Revillard JP, Owen E, Dubernard JM. Sequential histological and immunohistochemical study of the skin of the first human hand allograft. *Transplantation* 2000; 69: 1380-5.
8. Kanitakis J, Juillen D, Nicolas JF, De Boer B, Claudy A, Dubernard JM. Regeneration of cutaneous innervation in a human hand allograft. *Lancet* 2000; 356: 1738-9.
9. Gold BG, Yew JY, Zeleny-Pooley M. The immunosuppressant FK506 increases GAP-43 mRNA levels in axotomized sensory neurons. *Neurosci Lett* 1998; 241: 25-8.
10. Giraux P, Sirigu A, Schneider F, Dubernard JM. Cortical reorganization in motor cortex after graft of both hands. *Nature Neurosci* 2001; 4: 691-2.

The experience of three cases of human hand allografts in China

Guoxian Pei, Lijun Zhu, Liqiang Gu
Department of Orthopaedics & Traumatology, Nangfang Hospital, The First Military Medical University, Guangzhou, P. R. China

The first successful human hand transplantation was done at the Edouard Herriot Hospital in Lyon, France, on September 23, 1998 [1]; the second on January 24, 1999, in Louisville, Kentucky, USA [2]. In September 21, 1999, in Guangzhou, China, two human hand allografts were simultaneously completed [3]. In September 26, 2000, in Guangzhou, China, bilateral hand allografts were successfully transplanted. The three cases of human hand allograft are reported in the current paper. Three male recipients, with traumatic right wrist amputation of 2 years, were matched respectively to two ABO- and Rh-compatible (HLA compatibility: HLA-A, B, DR, DQ in case 1 and 2, HLA-A, B, DQ in case 3) brain-dead donors, direct crossmatch were performed to confirm the absence of prior sensitization to alloantigens. After amputation the donor's arm was irrigated with UW organ preservation solution at 4 °C, and transported in a box with ice. Three donor arms in case 1 and 3 were irradiated by 8gy X-ray before transplantation. The transplantation involved radial and ulnar bone fixation, anastomoses of radial and ulnar atery, sutures of median and ulnar and radial nerves, joining of tendons except flexors digitorum superficialis, and skin closure. After surgery the patients were given wide-spectrum antibiotics, anticoagulation and antispasm agents, and immunosuppressants, which included antithymocyte globins, FK506, mycophenolic acid, prednisone systematically and fluocinolone acetonide ointment locally. Clinical observations included vital signs and circulation of the hands. Immune state was monitored by assaying of C-reactive protein, Igs and PRA in the blood. Skin biopsy was done to exclude the dermal rejection. One of the patients developed venous crisis 1 hour postoperation. The exploratory operation found thrombosis in the cephalic vein, which was then removed and bridged by saphenous vein graft. Two of the patients developed hyperglycaemia, which required insulin administration. The skin healed and the sutures were removed 2 weeks postop. The nerve regeneration were found more rapid by Tinel's sign. The function of grafted hands recovered well. The present cases confirm that combination of currently available immunosupression agents can prevent acute rejection of human hand allograft and the tissues heal and the early function recover similarly to those in autologous replantation.

References

1. Dubernard JM, Oven E, Herzberg G. Human Hand allograft: report on first 6 months. *Lancet* 1999; 353: 1315-20.
2. Jones JW, Gruber SA, Barker JH, *et al.* Successful hand transplantation: one-year follow-up. *N Engl J Med* 2000; 343: 468-73.
3. A report of two cases of human hand allograft. *Nat Med J China* 2000; 80: 417-21.

Immunosupression in hand allograft

Nicole Lefrançois
Service de Transplantation, Hôpital Édouard-Herriot, Lyon, France

Experimental studies

The success of any composite tissue allografts (CTA), such as hand transplantation, depends on the prevention of rejection and several studies have demonstrated that each component of CTA interacts with the host immune system with a distinct degree of antigenicity and it is rejected by different mechanisms [1].

Most experimental studies [2, 3] have been performed in rodents. In this model a combination of several immunosuppressive drugs was required to prevent graft rejection. Indeed, using only one immunosuppressive drug, such as cyclosporine (CsA), long-term survival could not be achieved without major side effects. Experimental studies performed in rodents by Lee *et al.* [1, 4, 5] suggested that whole-limb allografts were less antigenic than grafts of each individual tissue. Several hypotheses were offered to explain this finding, including high antigenic load, antigenic competition, or the migration of donor leukocytes (dendritic cells). According to several experimental studies [1-8] the skin seems to be the most antigenic structure within a human CTA. In animal models [9] as well as in the clinical experience signs of skin rejection were not correlated with any other parameter.

More important information on CTA was provided by large animal [10] and primate models [11, 12] which present a closer analogy to the human immune system. Conversely in primates a very high level of immunosuppression was necessary to prevent rejection. In contrast all the human hand grafts remained viable with only conventional levels of immunosuppression.

The combination of FK506, mycophenolate mofetil (MMF) and prednisone as well as CsA/MMF/prednisone was shown to prolong graft survival in outbred swine models but no study has been performed using a combination immunosuppressant therapy in a primate model [13].

The Lyon team, which performed the first hand transplantation, decided to use as maintenance therapy a combination of agents which differ in mechanisms of action and toxicity profiles. The association FK506/MMF/prednisone was chosen because of its known efficacy in the swine model [14] and an apparent capacity of FK506 to accelerate axonal regeneration [15].

Immunosuppressive protocol

Induction therapy was used from several groups to avoid acute rejection. It can include polyclonal antibodies such as antithymocyte globulins and antilymphocyte globulins or monocolonal antibodies such as anti-CD 25 antibodies. We decide to use antithymocyte globulins as initial T lymphocyte depletion was considered to increase the effectiveness of maintenance therapy [16].

Maintenance therapy including FK506, MMF, prednisone is the association used in the majority of the cases of hand transplantation. This immunosuppressive protocol is comparable to that of organ transplantation with a similar rate of reconstitution of lymphocyte subsets and no evidence of overimmunosuppression. On the other side any reduction of immunosuppression is likely to carry a risk of rejection.

Adverse effects

Because of the adverse effects reported in experimental CTAs, particularly in primates [17], it seemed that the immunosuppression required for successful CTA would entail too high a risk of toxicity to justify clinical application. However, in the hand transplantations performed over the world the side effects related to treatment were limited to rapidly reversible serum sickness, transitory hyperglycemia, Herpes virus infection, CMV infection, Tinea infection, Cushing syndrome [18-21].

Tolerance, chimerism and graft-*versus*-host disease

Tolerance has not been demonstrated by any group [18-21].

Recipient's Langerhans cells were found by day 77 post-transplant only in the first grafted hand [22]. In rodent models CTAs that contain vascularized bone marrow can induce stable mixed chimerism and donor specific immunological tolerance as well as graft-*versus*-host-disease (GvHD), but the mechanisms underlying these events remain uncertain [9]. The possibility that both events might be extrapolated to human hand transplantation was considered, despite the low hematopoietic activity in adult human hand bones as compared with that of a young rat femur. Actually no signs of chimerism and/or GvHD were demonstrated in human hand transplantations [18-21].

Rejection episodes

Clinical and histological evaluation of the skin proved to be the only reliable parameter to identify rejection episodes. Acute rejection lesions were characterized by edema, erithema and maculo-papular lesions.

It is intriguing that, in contrast with primate models, acute rejection episodes in human hand allotransplantation can be completely reversed. Daniel et al. [23] and Stark et al. [24] reported a few reversals of acute rejection with very high CsA doses and corticosteroids. Stevens *et al.* [25] obtained similar results with monoclonal antibody therapy, but not with steroids alone.

In hand transplanted patients [18-21] acute rejection episodes were rapidly and completely reversed by steroids along with topical application of immunosuppressants. For the first time topical immunosuppressive drugs were employed showing to be efficacious.

The first hand grafted patient developed like-lichenoid lesions, which were considered as sign of chronic rejection.

In conclusion, the positive results obtained in the human hand transplantations performed over the world (France, USA, China, Austria, Italy) demonstrated that long-term viability is possible with the current immunosuppressive protocols used in solid organ transplantation. Rejection episodes can be monitored by clinical examination and skin biopsies and successfully treated by topical and systemic corticosteroid treatment. Although at present development of tolerance and GvHD were not seen and the immunosuppressive treatment was well supported, a longer follow-up will be necessary to evaluate the risk of chronic immunosuppression.

References

1. Lee WPA, Yaremchuk MJ, Pan YC, *et al.* Relative antigenicity of components of a vascularized limb allograft. *Plast Reconstr Surg* 1991; 87: 401-11.
2. Black KS, Hewitt CW, Fraser LA, *et al.* Composite tissue (limb) allografts in rats: I. Dose-dependent increase in survival with cyclosporine. *Transplantation* 1985; 39: 360-4.
3. Black KS, Hewitt CW, Hwang JS, Borger RW, Achauer BM. Dose response of cyclosporine-treated composite tissue allografts in a strong histoincompatible rat model. *Transpl Proc* 1988; 20 (Suppl. 2): 266-8.
4. Egerszegi EP, Samulack DD, Daniel RK. Experimental models in primates for reconstructive surgery utilizing tissue transplants. *Ann Plast Surg* 1984; 13: 423-30.
5. Gold ME, Randzio J, Kniha H, *et al.* Transplantation of vascularized composite mandibula allograft in young Cytomolgus monkeys. *Ann Plast Surg* 1991; 26: 125-32.
6. Hewitt CW. Update and outline of the experimental problems facing clinical composite tissue transplantation. *Transplant Proc* 1998; 30: 2704-7.
7. Lee WPA, Mathes DW. Hand transplantation: pertinent data and future outlook. *J Hand Surg* 1999; 24A: 906-13.
8. Llull R. An open proposal for clinical composite tissue allotransplantation. *Transplant Proc* 1998; 30: 2692-6.
9. Jensen JN, Mackinnon SE. Composite tissue allotransplantation: a comprehensive review of the literature – Part III. *J Reconstr Microsurgery* 2000; 16: 235-51.
10. Üstüner ET, Zdichavsky M, Ren X, *et al.* Long-term composite tissue allograft survival in a porcine model with cyclosporine/mycophenolate mofetil therapy. *Transplantation* 1998; 66: 1581-7.
11. Daniel RK, Egerszegi EP, Samulack DD, Skanes SE, Dykes RW, Rennie WRJ. Tissue transplants in primates for upper extremity reconstruction: a preliminary report. *J Hand Surg* 1986; 11A: 1-8.
12. Stark GB, Swartz WM, Narayanan K, Moller AR. Hand transplantation in baboons. *Transplant Proc* 1987; 19: 3968-71.
13. Jensen JN, Mackinnon SE. Composite tissue allotransplantation: a comprehensive review of the literature – Part II. *J Reconstr Microsurg* 2000; 16: 235-51.
14. Jones JW, Ustuner ET, Zdichavsky M, *et al.* Long-term survival of an extremity composite tissue allograft with FK 506-mycophenolate mofetil therapy. *Surgery* 1999; 126: 384-8.
15. Gold BG, Yew JY, Zeleny-Pooley M. The immunosuppressant FK506 increases GAP-43 mRNA levels in axotomized sensory neurons. *Neurosci Lett* 1998; 241: 25-8.

16. Preville X, Flacher M, LeMauff B, Beuchard S, Davelu P, Tioiller J, Revillard JP. Mechanism involved in antithymocyte globulin immunosuppressive activity in a nonhuman primate model. *Transplantation* 2001; 71: 460-8.
17. Stevens HPJD, Hovius SER, Heeney IL, van Nierop PW, Jonker M. Immunologic aspects of complications of composite tissue allografting for upper extremity reconstruction: a study in the rhesus monkey. *Transplant Proc* 1991; 23: 623-5.
18. Dubernard JM, Owen E, Herzberg G, Lanzetta M, Martin X, Kapila H, Dawahra M, Hakim NS. Human hand allograft: report on first 6 months. *Lancet* 1999; 353: 1315-20.
19. Dubernard JM, Owen E, Lefrancois N, Petruzzo P, Martin X, Dawahra M, Juillen D, Kanitakis J, Frances C, Preville X, Gebuhrer L, Hakim N, Lanzetta M, Kapila H, Herzberg G, Revillard JP. First human hand transplantation. *Transpl Int* 2000; 13: 521-4.
20. Jones JW, Gruber SA, Barker JH, Breindenbach WC. Successful hand transplantation: one year follow-up. *New Engl J Med* 2000; 343: 468-73.
21. Francois CG, Bredeinbach WC, Maldonado C, Kakoulidis TP, Hodges A, Dubernard JM, Owen E, Pei G, Ren X, Barker JH. Hand transplantation: comparison and observations of the first four clinical cases. *Microsurgery* 2000; 20: 360-71.
22. Kanitakis J, Juillen D, Nicolas JF, Frances C, Claudy A, Revillard JP, Owen E, Dubernard JM. Sequential histological and immunohistochemical study of the skin of the first human hand allograft. *Transplantation* 2000; 69: 1380-5.
23. Daniel RK, Egerszegi EP, Samulack DD, Skanes SE, Dykes RW, Rennie WR. Tissue transplants in primates of upper extremity reconstruction: a preliminary report. *J Hand Surg* 1986; 11: 1-8.
24. Stark GB, Swartz WM, Narayanan R, Moller A. Hand transplantation in baboons. *Transplant Proc* 1987; 19: 3968-71.
25. Stevens HPJD, Hovius SER, Vuzevski VD, et al. Immunological aspects of allogeneic partial hand transplantation in the rhesus monkey. *Transplant Proc* 1990; 22: 2006-8.

Composite Tissue Allografts
Dubernard J.-M., ed.
© John Libbey Eurotext, Paris, 2001

Bilateral hand transplant: functional results after 18 months

Bernard Vallet[1], Hélène Parmentier[2], Valérie Lagouy[1], Natacha Dziesmiazkiewiez[1]

[1] Centre de réadaptation fonctionnelle le Val-Rosay, Saint-Didier-au-Mont-d'Or, France
[2] Hôpital Édouard-Herriot, Lyon, France

There are three challenges involved in re-education following a bilateral hand transplant. First, guaranteeing that there is a result that is comparable with that of the standard reimplantation of an upper limb in terms of both motricity and sensitivity. Secondly, obtaining autonomy that is at least equivalent to that of prostheses and technical aids. And thirdly, responding in terms of restoring body image to an aspect of the request for a transplant that is very complex in this type of patient.

In this article we report our experiences in the evolution of sensitivity, motricity and autonomy after 18 months in the first patient to receive a bilateral hand transplant.

The overall results are comparable between the right and left hand, even though progress has not been totally symmetrical. It has not been possible to distinguish from this what is the result of the surgery and what comes from the patient's previous laterality.

From a sensorial point of view, our patient has acquired sensitivity to pricking and temperature, as well as sensitivity to pressure from a Semmes-Weinstein 4.56 mono filament. This protection sensitivity mainly concerns the palmar surfaces and the entire digital pulp regions.

Discriminatory sensitivity is still poor (Moberg TP test and Dellon MTP test greater than or equal to 15 mm). This type of recuperation is marked by the existence of errors in analyzing movement direction as well as in perception of spatial representation with confusion in areas of proximity.

Tactile recognition of large, everyday objects (such as a lighter, pen, keys or eraser) was obtained easily in the bi-manual mode, but has been more difficult for delicate objects (such as buttons, paper clips and matches). In addition, we have noted that there is acquisition of mental recognition of forms and objects beyond any prior presentation. Geometric shapes (square, rectangle, diamond, circle and so on) are recognized by palming the object or by following the contours without moving the forearms.

Textures that are rough or intermediary are recognized easily (sandpaper, hessian, felt and velvet) with an average reflection time of 15 seconds.

The mobility of the wrists and fingers is good with the fingers almost completely able to unfurl and roll up passively. Active mobility is limited by muscle tension caused by adherence, but the patient is able to bring his thumb and index finger into contact and his thumb and middle finger close together.

Extrinsic muscular force is of good quality, measured at between 4 and 5. It remains poor for most of the intrinsic muscles, indicating that reinnervation is not symmetrical and is still incomplete for the median and ulnar nerves on both sides. Active rolling of the fingers remains incomplete because of major dyssynergia between the extrinsic flexor muscles and the activity of the lumbricales muscles with a pulp-palm distance of 3 cm.

The current deficit in the thenar muscles does not enable the patient to obtain any real thumb-index opposition.

For this reason, functional gestures remain essentially of the subterminal-lateral type, with a maximum force of 600 mg.

There is some difficulty in holding spherical or cylindrical objects. Holding delicate objects (such as a needle) or objects that require physical force (using a screwdriver) remains unsatisfactory.

The patient can pick up, using a hook movement, a weight of more than 8 kg.

In comparison to the autonomy of the patient before the operation, the gain in autonomy has been significant in terms of all elementary everyday activities, including hygiene, dressing, eating, household and occupational tasks. A certain number of tasks that were previously impossible have been acquired (writing, using scissors, carrying weight) or simplified by the elimination of the need for technical aids (opening jars, using a zipper, using a mobile telephone).

In opposition to persistently using two hands for simple gestures (which probably comes from the residual memory of using stumps), the appearance of automatic and quick one-handed gestures has been noted, suggesting that there is cortical integration when sensorimotor information is processed.

This evolution will be encouraged by continuing sensitivity recuperation and work in dissociation with the fingers.

In comparison to a standard reimplantation, this bilateral hand allograft has produced encouraging results after 18 months. The gain in autonomy, through recuperation of sensitivity and motricity already obtained, is beneficial for the patient and reassures him in his treatment choice.

In the longer term, assessing this type of reimplantation will, on the condition that there is a complementary series of questions, raises just one question: when should the transplant be performed?

The quality of the final result is effectively partially dependent on the amount of time that passes between the initial amputation and the reimplantation, for both anatomical reasons (atrophy of the stumps) and cortical reasons (loss of the memorization of acquisitions).

Cortical reorganisation after hand transplantation

Pascal Giraux[1,2], Angela Sirigu[1], Fabien Schneider[3], Jean-Michel Dubernard[4]

[1] *Institute for Cognitive Science, CNRS, Bron, France*
[2] *Department of Physical Medicine, CHU, Saint-Étienne, France*
[3] *Radiology Department, CHU, Saint-Étienne, France*
[4] *Department of Surgical Transplant, E. Herriot Hospital, Lyon, France*

Among the wide network of brain regions devoted to the motor control, some of them, including the primary motor cortex and the primary sensitive cortex, seem to be organised as maps of adjacent body segments. These maps have been initially described as "homunculus" by Penfield [1], and in the last two decades, their modelisation has evolved from a rather fixed and clear-cut organisation to a highly plastic mosaic of body segments [2]. A high degree of plasticity have been shown in varied situations including nerve lesions [3], spinal cord injury [4], brain injury [5] and limb amputation.

In the present case of amputation, the representation of the unaffected adjacent body segments expands so that the representation of the stump region invades portions of the sensorimotor cortex previously dedicated to the amputated segment [6, 7]. In such patients, the absence of a limb may lead to strong phantom sensations accompanied in some cases by pain [8]. The painful feeling seems to be positively correlated with the degree of cortical reorganisation present in the sensorimotor cortex [9]. In non-human primates with accidental or therapeutic amputation of the digits or the forearm, intracortical stimulation of the motor cortex (M1) in the region corresponding to the missing segment yields muscular contractions in the stump and in neighbouring areas [10]. A system of horizontal connections in the sensorimotor cortex, in particular in layers II, III and in the collateral of layer V pyramidal cells could account for the extension of the motor and sensory representations of the adjacent body segments after nerve lesions or amputation [11].

Patients who received transplantation of the upper limb following their amputation are questioning the reversibility of the cerebral reorganisation. By the mean of functional MRI, we investigated the nature and time-course of cortical rearrangement of the body motor representation produced by hand allograft [12].

Methods

Patient's clinical data

CD is a 33 year-old right-handed gardener who sustained a traumatic amputation of both hands in 1996, 3 cm above wrists. The patient wore daily two myoelectrical prosthesis, which allowed a bilateral pinch grip. Before transplantation he experienced bilateral painless phantom limb sensations, with a subjective ability to "move" easily and independently all digits. The phantom was so vivid that he could even "count" all digits. When instructed to perform a flexion and an extension of the "four fingers", corresponding extrinsic muscles contractions in the forearms were evident through simple palpation of the stump. The first 6 weeks following transplantation, no active movement was allowed. Two months after transplantation, CD was able to partially flex together the 4 last digits of both hands, but was unable to produce extension movements. At 4 and 6 months, the ability to flex and extend together the 4 last digits progressively increased, although differentiated digit movements were impossible. At 6 months post-surgery, the patient could perform a bilateral partial pinch grip. Somatic sensations also partially recovered. Pressure and temperature sensitivity was evident in the palm and dorsum at 4 months, and at the extremity of all digits at 6 months. Detection of simple tactile stimuli applied to both the palm and the dorsum of the hands was impossible at 2 months although the patient's performance greatly improved at 4 and 6 months.

Material and procedure

We performed four identical fMRI examinations, the first 6 months before the graft and three post-operatively: 2, 4 and 6 months after the graft. We used a 1 Tesla Siemens MRI machine, EPI sequence, Repetition Time = 5.3 sec, 18 slices 3.5×3.5 mm in-plane resolution, 6 mm width, 4 sessions per examination, 110 scans per session. We used an event-related fMRI paradigm with regularly spaced events (26 sec = 5 scans). The task required the patient to perform flexion/extension of the last four digits of the left or right hand and flexion/extension of the left or right elbow. In the pre-surgery exam and the first post-surgery exam, flexion and extension of the fingers were impossible and were monitored through palpation of the corresponding extrinsic muscle contractions at the level of the forearm. The analysis was performed using SPM99 software (Wellcome Department of Cognitive Neurology, London, UK). EPI data were convolved with a standard Hemodynamic Response Flow Model. The statistical T-maps were calculated on the remaining variance. For each condition we chose a corrected threshold at $p < 0.05$ corresponding to a $Z = 5.07$. Statistical comparisons between conditions were performed with an uncorrected threshold at $p < 0.001$ ($Z = 3.1$) and with an additional spatial extend threshold at $p < 0.05$. An inclusive statistical mask constituted by the activations of the positive component was used during comparisons of independent examinations (*e.g.* pre-surgery minus 6 months). Cluster size is reported in the T1 MRI resolution ($2 \times 2 \times 2$ mm). The center of gravity of M1 activations was calculated in both the hand and elbow conditions using the Z-score of each activated voxel as a weighting parameter. The study was approved by the local Ethical Comity (Centre Léon Bérard).

Results

Our analysis mainly focused on the activations in the primary motor cortex and their evolution over time. In the pre-surgery exam, movements of both the right and the left hand activated the most lateral part of the hand area in M1. Six months after the graft, the hand representation expanded medially and occupied the entire hand region, including some of the pre-surgery activation. Direct statistical comparison between the first (pre-surgery) and last (6 months) examinations indicated that lateral M1 sites that were active for hand movements prior to the graft were less active following the graft, and that a medial site that was not active before became active after the graft *(Table I)*. The time course of this displacement was illustrated by the evolution of the center of gravity (COG) of M1 activations. Across the four examinations, COG of hand activations showed a progressive shift of 10 mm for the right hand and 6 mm for the left hand from the lateral to the central part of the hand region *(Table II)*.

Table I. Comparison between pre-surgery and 6 months examinations

	Pre-surg. minus 6 months			6 months minus pre-surg		
	COG x y z (mm)	Z-score	Cluster size	COG x y z (mm)	Z-score	Cluster size
Right hand	- 43 - 19 38	5.5	58	- 24 - 34 57	5.4	26
Left hand	36 - 19 46	> 10	288	27 - 28 56	8.5	55
Right elbow	- 38 - 24 43	5.3	112	- 14 - 38 56	5	37
Left elbow	32 - 22 46	> 10	220	26 - 27 57	8.6	86

COG = center of gravity.

Table II. Time-course of the center of gravity of M1 activations for the hand and elbow and for the different exams

Movement	Pre-surg. x y z	2 months x y z	4 months x y z	6 months x y z	Distance Pre-surg. → 6 months
Right hand	- 42 - 22 40	- 40 - 25 46	- 39 - 25 45	- 39 - 27 48	10 mm
Left hand	36 - 18 46	33 - 23 49	38 - 21 48	33 - 22 49	6 mm
Right elbow	- 34 - 29 49	- 26 - 33 54	- 30 - 31 52	- 28 - 32 54	8 mm
Left elbow	31 - 23 47	29 - 28 51	30 - 26 52	30 - 26 54	7 mm

Talairach's co-ordinates.

Elbow movements produced a pattern of motor activations which evolved in time in parallel with the hand motor representation. Before surgery, movements of either elbow triggered an extensive activation in a contralateral central region of M1, corresponding to the hand motor map. At 6 months post-surgery, elbow activations migrated toward an area situated in the upper part of the limb representation and classically defined as the arm region. Statistical comparison between the first (pre-surgery) and last (6 months) examinations demonstrated that different M1 cortical maps were associated to the pre-surgery and post-surgery period: a more central region before the graft, and a new superior medial area 6 months after the graft. The time course of the COGs along the four examinations indicated a progressive shift from the central to the superior part of M1 being of 8 mm for the right elbow and 7 mm for the left elbow *(Table I)*.

The changes observed within the motor cortex for hand and elbow representations appeared to be strongly correlated not only in time but also in space. Across the different examinations the distance between COGs remained fairly constant for the two types of movements (right hand, right elbow: pre-surgery = 14 mm, 2 months = 13 mm, 4 months = 13 mm, 6 months = 12 mm; left hand, left elbow: pre-surgery = 7 mm, 2 months = 10 mm, 4 months = 10 mm, 6 months = 7 mm). Interestingly, in the pre-surgery period the COG co-ordinates for elbow activations were situated near by the spatial co-ordinates observed for the COG of hand movement at 6 months *(Table II)*. It should also be noted that hand and elbow activations showed a high degree of overlap.

Parallel to the motor cortex modifications, changes were also recorded in the somatosensory cortex. Hand movements activated S1 in all four examinations. Before surgery, right hand activations were found laterally just behind and adjacent to the activated motor region. Post-surgery, parallel displacements from lateral to medial sites were observed in both M1 and S1. Analysis of the S1 COGs between the pre-surgery and the 6 months post-surgery exams showed a shift of 10 mm. Changes were also observed for elbow movements and their pattern follow the one observed in the case of motor cortex activations.

Discussion

These results show that a bilateral hand allograft has a direct effect on the hand and elbow representations in the sensorimotor cortex. The displacement of the cortical activity from lateral to medial along the precentral gyrus is remarkably similar for both hand and elbow movements. These cortical maps covered in the same amount of time a similar distance, as revealed by the trajectory of the activation COGs. This suggests that new peripheral inputs allow a global remodelling of the limb cortical map and reverse the functional reorganisation induced by the amputation. The spatial trajectory of these activations in time further indicates that the cortical rearrangement takes place in an orderly way: the hand and arm representations tend to return to their original cortical locus.

References

1. Penfield W. *The cerebral cortex of the man*. New York: MacMillan, 1950.
2. Sanes JN, Donoghue JP. Plasticity and primary motor cortex. *Annu Rev Neurosci* 2000; 23: 393-415.
3. Sanes JN. Dynamic organization of primary motor cortex output to target muscles in adult rats. I. Long-term patterns of reorganization following motor or mixed peripheral nerve lesions. *Exp Brain Res* 1990; 79 (3): 479-91.
4. Topka H. Reorganization of corticospinal pathways following spinal cord injury. *Neurology* 1991; 41: 1276-83.
5. Rossini PM. Hand motor cortical area reorganization in stroke: a study with fMRI, MEG and TCS maps. *Neuroreport* 1998; 9: 2141-6.
6. Roricht S, Meyer BU. Residual function in motor cortex contralateral to amputated hand. *Neurology* 2000; 54: 984-7.
7. Cohen LG, et al. Motor reorganization after upper limb amputation in man. A study with focal magnetic stimulation. *Brain* 1991; 114: 615-27.
8. Ramachandran VS. The perception of phantom limbs. *Brain* 1998; 121: 1603-30.

9. Flor H, et al. Phantom-limb pain as a perceptual correlate of cortical reorganization following arm amputation. *Nature* 1995; 375: 482.
10. Qi HX, Stepniewska I, Kaas JH. Reorganization of primary motor cortex in adult macaque monkeys with long-standing amputations. *J Neurophysiol* 2000; 84: 2133.
11. Huntley GW. Correlation between patterns of horizontal connectivity and the extend of short-term representational plasticity in rat motor cortex. *Cereb Cortex* 1997; 7: 143-56.
12. Giraux P, Sirigu A, Schneider F, Dubernard JM. Cortical reorganization in motor cortex after graft of both hands. *Nature Neurosci* 2001; 4 (7): 691-2.

Indications for hand allografts

M. Lanzetta
Hand Surgery and Reconstructive Microsurgery Unit, University of Milan-Bicocca, Italy

Selection of the ideal patient is the most important issue in hand transplantation. Strict criteria must be applied to select the candidates to this procedure. Selection must involve a collegial evaluation of the patient involving not only the surgeons, but also the physicians, a clinical psychologist, an immunologist, a hand therapist, an anaesthesiologist, a lawyer, and the patient's general practitioner. At the moment, we recommend the following inclusion criteria: age comprised between 18 and 50 years, traumatic amputation, dominant hand or bilateral at the wrist level, tried and refused different prosthetic alternatives, otherwise healthy and mentally sane, able to give an informed consent, resident in the country, available to follow-up.

Two kinds of patients are not good candidates: lower limb amputees and congenital amputees. Lower limbs have a different "value" and function compared to upper limbs. Their main function is to permit weight bearing and ambulation. They do not have additional functions in terms of social and emotional interactions with others, nor have a strong symbolic value. Current prosthetic solutions absolve well the task of stability, weight bearing and walk. Clothes can easily disguise them, so that they are not apparent to the others. At this stage the benefit of a living transplanted leg does not outweight the drawbacks of current immunosuppressive therapy complications.

In the case of congenital amputations and malformations, we do not yet know enough. In these cases the missing part has never been lost, but simply has never been there. This means that no information has been transferred from the absent part to the brain, and no commands have been imparted to it. Although it would be logical to conclude that the cortical representation of this part is missing, there is some evidence that this might not be the case. This relates mainly to the incidence of phantom limb in congenital (aplasic) absence of limbs. Aplasic phantoms are based on the existence of specific neural circuitry associated with innate motor schemas, such as the neural matrix responsible for early hand-mouth coordination. It is therefore hypothesized that the neural network, or "neuromatrix", that subserves body sensation has a genetically determined substrate that is modified by sensory experience. If transplanted from a donor, nerves would probably advance in the allograft, given the tremendous potential for regeneration in children. Would they then transfer meaningful data to the central nervous system and in which area? The clinical experience with toe-to-hand transfers in congenital cases confirms that cortical plasticity allows for complete integration of the added part. Therefore, it might be hypothesized that composite tissue allografts for reconstruction of congenital malformations should be performed very early to accommodate for the greater capacity of integration.

The psychiatrist and the hand transplant

Danièle Bachman, Gabriel Burloux
Hôpital Édouard-Herriot, Lyon, France

Our subject is the psychical assessment of patients before the transplant of either one or two hands, as performed in Lyons, France, and the follow-up of these patients.

Psychical assessment

The ethical point of view

There are ethical concerns about this kind of graft. There is no vital need for the operation as is the case with heart or liver transplants. One could say there is no vital need either in kidney or pancreas transplants, the life of the patient not being at stake as there are other means (dialysis, insulin treatment) which are cumbersome but allow the patient to stay alive.

In the case of hand transplants, we have to assess accurately in terms of quality of life the benefit provided by the graft, as opposed to the use of an artificial limb.

In France, the Comité d'Éthique now prohibits the transplantation of only one hand if the other is valid, because the handicap is deemed not important enough compared to the constraints involved.

Pre-graft psychical assessment

Interviews

Clinical interviews, performed by psyche specialists are of crucial importance, and even extremely useful if performed by two of them. Indeed, it allows a richer confrontation of views. Different issues are to be assessed:

1. How the patient understands the absolute necessity of the immunosuppressive treatment, and the risks (infections, cancers, rejection, and possibly amputation) and side-effects (diabetes, overweight, etc.) associated with it.

2. How the patient will go through such a heavy operation, the pain and the dependency after the graft. Indeed, he will find himself in a even worse situation than before the operation.

3. How the patient will succeed in carrying out physiotherapy and will be able to regularly take his treatment in the long run.

4. Motivation and determination:

– Is the mourning for the lost hands over, *i.e.* is there a relative acceptance of the lost object, never easy to achieve? For instance, our two patients were convinced that they will one day have their hands back (which was an impossible thing at the time). It shows that the mourning phase was not over.

– Narcissistic and functional motivations:

• The rationale for the graft can be of a narcissistic nature: the patient wants to restore the self-image that was maimed, suffering from the way others look at him, perceived as deprecating and pitiful.

• Recovering motricity and sensitivity is the other part of the motivation in order to regain autonomy and a better relationship with people around thanks to the graft. Of course, both types of motivations exist. The more functional they are, the better it is. Indeed, it is a predictive factor of how the patient will endure all the constraints, side-effects and physiotherapy, as mentioned before.

5. Idealization

This is a very important dimension to evaluate as there is an unavoidable disappointment in terms of what the patient is actually able to do compared to what he expected. Indeed, what he wants is to be "as before". The greatest is the difference between what the patient had imagined and the reality he has to go through after the graft, the greatest is his disappointment. The difficult process of mourning over the hands is followed by mourning over the delusions linked with the graft. Hence a risk of depression, a disinvolvement in physiotherapy, an unability to support the constraints associated with the treatment, including putting an end to the treatment.

Idealization is both narcissistic (to regain a good body image) and functional (to be able to recover former abilities, like playing the piano, driving a car, etc.) Moreover, the time needed for a satisfactory recovery may last for one to two years. There is a specificity attached to this transplant. What is expected when a kidney, liver or heart is grafted is that it works (it works or it doesn't work). In this case, the doctor and the patient share the same point of view. In the case of a hand transplant, the doctor may be happy with a result that will not satisfy the patient.

6. Traumatophilia

Losing hands is traumatic. The transplantation of hands is also traumatic both physically and psychologically (from a psychical point of view). As a matter of fact, there are people who are accident-prone or "traumatophilic" as psycho-analysts say. It is very important to assess this propensity for having accidents as those people are liable to repetition (which was true for our two patients). It is also important to assess the part of the trauma that has not been integrated in the mind or elaborated upon before the operation. The greater it is, the bigger the risk of hallucinatory recall of the trauma (for instance in the post-op days).

7. The patient's personality and possible psychiatric troubles

In sum, these interviews aim to identify factors in favour of the operation and other aspects that might work against it and to weigh their respective importance.

– *Factors in favour of the operation*

- The determination and enthusiasm shown by the patient to undergo the graft (which was a risky adventure not so long ago and even now). We may know about it from what the patient has done in his life before the graft and his ability to project himself into the future (considering the length of physiotherapy and the scope of all the expectations: aesthetics, functionality, sensitivity, etc.) and the relative irreversibility of the process.

- The patient's ability to regress. On the one hand, regression is an absolute necessity but on the other hand it must not go too far and last too long (as it would turn into depression). What is important is the "quality" of that regression and the psychiatrist has to check on it.

– *Negative factors*

- While the positive factors are fairly apparent, these are largely unconscious. The conditions, details and images of the accident which were more or less repressed or denied come back with force to the mind insomuch as the conditions that prevailed after the accident look like the post-op days of the amputation (bandages, nursing, pain, immobility, etc.). A post-traumatic neurosis may be reactivated with nightmares, visual images of the earlier accident, along with hallucinations. This is to be foreseen before the graft.

- Fantasizing about the cadaver. A grafted hand comes from a cadaver: it is not functional and the sight of it is rather terrible (colour, stitches, blood, etc.). The idea is that something from a corpse is joined to a living body, and this echoes an old human fantasy (Frankenstein). This hand could go back to its former cadaveric state and it is somewhat alien and so could live its proper life and do things against the will of the receiver inasmuch as the latter has no motor control of the hand (the "Adams Family" syndrome). Those fantasies, including the idea of crime, are to be repressed, especially if they are close to unconscious desires (!).

- The question of the donor implies a necessary denial to endure the sight of this dead graft. This does not prevent the receiver from having a feeling of debt and guilt (as though the donor had died because of him) and also of gratitude and identification with some qualities or defaults of the latter.

Tests

We have used a certain number of tests, namely Minimult which assesses the patient's personality and is replicable throughout the follow-up process. The results confirmed the clinical evaluation. Other possible tests are: MMPI II, Rorschach or TAT which allow a better assessment as far as the body image is concerned.

The family circle

Our experience showed how important the feelings and reactions of the family circle are. What is true for the patient is also true for the family (hand deemed as that of a corpse, non-functionality, etc.). Moreover, if the family doesn't live in the city where the graft is performed, the patient cannot share with them all the difficulties and pain he goes through, so that they end up living in two different worlds. It should be added that the hand is a tool for contact and relation with a symbolic and social aspect to it, mainly with the family. It is a factor of autonomy for the person and it allows exchanges with others, including sexual relations.

Even though everybody in the family circle wants the patient to recover sufficient autonomy and escape the dependency he suffered before the graft, how do they accept this new hand, which is dead, strange and alien, slowly coming back to life in such an odd way? Proper acceptance of the graft by the people around him is very helpful in the process of "taming" the transplanted hands. Their reaction furthers the inevitable and necessary psychological movements of denial, denial of the origin and of the unpleasant appearance of the hand. So the patient and the family are able to gradually integrate together in their minds all the aspects of the new hands. And this prevents questions like "did the donor die?" that halt the process of denial.

Follow-up

The framework

Patients are seen every day, sometimes more if something happens (delusion, anxiety, crisis) at the beginning and then less and less often, depending on how the case evolves.

As far as possible, we get in touch with the patient's family and social environment of the patient.

The whole medical team meets together once a week. Doctors exchange their point of view.

The post-op days and possible psychical disorders

1. Anxiety

As this type of graft can be described as "visible", anxiety in this case takes the form of de-personalization. It is linked to the alien nature of the grafted hand, its cadaveric aspect but also to the apparent boundary between the receiver's arm and the donor's hand, symbolic of a troublesome coexistence of the dead and the living, between the familiar and the unfamiliar.

This type of anxiety usually occurs right after the operation, and more so with the first bandages, but fails to be expressed as such: it can take the form of vagal disorders or of any kind of physical trouble, or even a recurrence of acute pain. It can last in a fluctuant manner until the psychological process of appropriation of the grafted hands is completed and firmly anchored.

The anxiety is in fact pre-existent to the graft and linked with the horror induced by the idea of mix or coexistence, or even of confusion between the living and the dead. With the first bandages, it is crystallized as a fear when the patient is faced with the vision of a dead hand hanging from his healthy elbow. That vision makes us remember our state of mortal beings.

2. Regression

It is a necessary and desirable step, at least to a certain extent, especially in the immediate aftermath of the transplantation when the patient is extremely dependent and back in a state in which he has few of the functional abilities he had gained before the graft using his stumps or prostheses. This regression is temporary and should not last too long in order not to prevent active physiotherapy. It goes with an operating mode in which the body becomes a privileged vehicle for the patient's anxiety and in which thought goes animistic, with fantasies of the hand taking on a life of its own and doing things beyond the patient's control.

3. Depression

As with idealization, it is a risk that is dependent on the possible fragile personality of the patient, but also on the necessary discrepancy between how the patient imagines his life after the graft and what he is able to perform in the real world. As we said, the greater the difference between the two, the greater the risk of depression.

4. Multi-factor delirium

Post-operative shock, steroid therapy, serum reactions or a reaction of the native hand against the grafted one are elements that can induce a confusional type of delirium. The risk is even more acute in the first post-op days, and compounded by a certain number of factors linked with the personality of the patient and by the reactivation of the initial trauma, which seems quite frequent.

5. Reactivation of the initial trauma which caused the loss of the hands

The post-op conditions remind the patient of the trauma and the circumstances after the accident: the bandages on the forearms (even though the tip of the fingers is visible after the transplant, which of course is not the case after the amputation), the regression associated with the state of total dependency as for all the ordinary gestures of everyday life (right after the transplant, the patient is absolutely unable to make use of the new hands attached to his forearms, and finds himself in a state of even greater dependency than just before the transplant, especially when the patient has learnt to master the use of his artificial limbs).

It is at that time that certain psychological phenomena may reappear, if they had disappeared in the first place: they are then reactivated acutely, under the form of visual "flashes" of the initial accident, anxiety, nightmares reliving the accident, etc.

However, enduring dependency throughout the period between the initial accident and the possible use of prostheses and the associated state of regression can make the adaptation period after the transplant somewhat easier.

6. Denial in the face of "alien" hands: splitting

This is probably what was the most surprising phenomenon for us, in particular because of its length and its fluctuating acuteness. Denial can be defined as a lack of perception of certain features of reality, or in lesser acute cases, as a perception of reality that is immediately negated or rejected. We were able to observe this denial as early as the first post-op days, to the point that one of the patients said that his own hands were grafted back. It is indeed a psychic defence mechanism put in place to keep at a distance the frightening perception of transplanted hands, with the violence linked to it that the psyche is unable to assimilate. As the new grafted hands gained in sensitivity and dexterity, the denial tended to lessen, and ten months later, the patient was able to evoke the donor and the "alien" nature of the hands, whereas he had succeeded in making them his own or, in other terms, in "taming" them thanks to physiotherapy, psychical follow-up and the increasingly better motor control of his hands.

One of the characteristics of denial is to return to the former state in a violent or even traumatic way, through the environment, that is to say through the comments made by the others (family, nurses and doctors, media) which insist on the morbid feeling to be facing a human being with dead hands attached. What is denied inside comes back from the outside.

Most of the time, denial goes with splitting: a mechanism whereby the person has two contradictory thoughts without perceiving the contradiction. In the case of hand transplants, it is therefore possible to think the hands are those of the patient or those of the dead donor. The two thoughts are concomitant in the patient's mind (patient, family circle, carers) but the antagonism is not an issue. Splitting is necessary in this particular condition, it makes it possible to take into account the two troublesome aspects of the hand transplant: hands taken from a dead body which, if everything goes well, will be back to life and become the hand of the receiver.

Splitting exist both in the patient's mind (he thinks the hand is both his and another person's) and in the carers' minds. As long as the two ideas remain separate, splitting allows the person to live with two contradictory thoughts. Unfortunately, this is never the case: the two thoughts often collide, the split breaks down and anxiety reappears. The denial then no longer works (examples include the sight of a patient biting his fingernails, the feeling of a too cold hand, the words: "I don't shake hands with a corpse" said to the patient).

Perspectives

The insight gained from following these two patients raise a host of other questions: it appears that the two patients' personality is rather particular, as both volunteered for an adventure whose outcome is uncertain. The pre-transplant assessment will probably be refined, in terms of interviews as well as tests. More than a psychiatric or psychical assessment, it should be a comprehensive assessment of the person taking into account his relationship with his family, friends and carers.

Hand transplants pave the way for other composite tissue allografts, for which the intervention of psyche specialists will be important, more so because of the visibility of this type of graft, absent in internal organ transplants.

The benefits for patients are still rather hard to quantify, but should in any case be set against their previous quality of life.

We are happy to have been at the outset of what seemed to be an adventure and which, without being a routine, is getting now more easily feasible.

Ethics

Composite Tissue Allografts
Dubernard J.-M., ed.
© John Libbey Eurotext, Paris, 2001

Composite tissue allografts: the donor side

Didier Houssin, Michel Bouvier d'Yvoire, Bernard Loty
Établissement français des greffes, Paris, France

The recent development of composite tissue allografts (CTAs), such as hand allografts, in man raises multiple medical, scientific and ethical questions with regard to the recipient. No less important questions are also raised on the donor side, since it is clear that the performance of such allografts implies the removal of the graft from the body of a recently deceased person. Such questions deserve close attention, not only for their consequences for the family of the deceased, but also for the hospital workers in charge of organ harvesting, and potentially through their impact on organ donation, for the patients waiting for a life-supporting organ.

Such attention is essential, if one considers that encouraging results of hand allografts might stimulate their practice and that future developments might extend the field of composite tissue allografts to even more controversial domains such as the allografts of male sexual organs or the whole human face.

Definition and recent history of CTAs

CTAs do not include any specific tissue or organ, and can be defined as "a vascularised allograft consisting of a composite of distinct tissues, predominantly of integumentary/musculoskeletal types, which potentially would be used for functional and cosmetic restoration of patients with severe tissue loss" [1, 2].

Before the first widely publicised hand allograft took place in Lyon in October 1998, allografts corresponding to the above definition of CTAs had already been performed, in particular three cases of vascularised femoral diaphysis allografts [3], three cases of vascularised total knee joint allografts [3], one case of muscular allograft for scalp reconstruction [4], numerous cases of nerve allografts [5], and two cases of complete digital flexion system (tendon/paratendon) vascularised allografts [6].

In June 2001, eight patients had undergone unilateral (six patients) or bilateral (two patients) hand allograft: two cases in Lyon (one bilateral), one case in Austria (bilateral), two cases in the United States of America and three cases in China. These patients are being actively followed-up. Follow-up data of the two French patients [7-12] and of the first US patient [13] have been published, as well as a summary of the experience gained with the first four cases [14].

Lastly, the observation of the first apparently successful laryngeal allograft was reported in May 2001 [15].

Is there a future for composite tissue allografts?

The potential CTAs indications which we are going to briefly discuss are: hand allografts, laryngeal allografts, complex CTAs for the reconstruction of major facial defects, and male external genital organs allografts.

Hand allografts

Hands are needed for almost every activity of daily living, are critical for communication and for the sense of touch, and are an essential part of our appearance. The loss of a hand or forearm is thus a devastating event, especially if bilateral.

Hand allografts, or rather upper limb extremity allografts, may be medically and ethically justified in patients who have a poor functional result with reconstructive surgery or prosthetic replacement techniques, especially if the amputation is bilateral, provided that i) sustained satisfactory function of the grafted hands is achievable, and ii) the overall costs to the patient (taking into account in particular the risks linked to immunosuppression) remain acceptable. It is therefore indispensable to assess in carefully designed clinical trials whether, in selected patients, the risk/benefit ratio is in favour of carrying out hand allografts. Such a clinical study of five cases of bilateral hand allograft is underway in France, with Dubernard as main investigator. Communication has been set up between the few teams who have undertaken to explore this pioneering technique, in order to share optimally the knowledge gained from the individual experience of each patient. Among the most interesting results already obtained are the post-graft motor and sensorimotor cortex modifications, suggesting that, contrary to the fears of some specialists, a good recovery of the long unused cortical areas may be possible even several years after amputation [12].

Laryngeal allografts

The report of the first apparently successful laryngeal allograft [15] shows that the première was done nearly at the same time, in 1998, as the première of the hand allograft, which suggests that the state of the art was at that time "ripe" for such complex CTAs. In this observation, it is interesting to note that, similarly to the cases of hand allografts: i) the rejection episodes could be well controlled with reasonable immunosuppression; ii) reinnervation of the graft took place satisfactorily and rapidly; iii) the delicate motor command of the larynx and pharynx could be recovered even though the allograft took place 20 years after the initial destructive trauma. Possibly the use of an electrolarynx partly helped to preserve the phonation nervous command potential.

The authors propose as potential candidates for laryngeal allografts aphonic patients with laryngeal trauma, patients with large benign chondromas requiring laryngectomy, and patients who have undergone laryngectomy for cancer and who remain disease-free after five years.

Reconstructive surgery for complex, extensive facial defects

Important facial destructions or malformations have extremely severe consequences, and can lead to a total or near total withdrawal of the patients from any form of social interaction. In the cases where traditional reconstructive surgery is either technically impossible or has failed, the extent of the disability of these patients may also justify the recourse to CTAs. Potential indications could include (Lantieri, personal communication): i) some cases of massive facial malformations; ii) some cases of severe neurofibromatosis; iii) massive facial traumas, such as can be seen in some cases of failed suicide using gunshot; iv) scalp avulsion when replantation is impossible or has failed.

No data are available yet on the actual incidence of such cases, which is probably low.

Male external genital organs

Testicular defects are usually dealt with using plastic surgery and hormone substitution. As for allotransplantation of the penis, potential indications can be theoretically considered, in particular congenital abnormalities (complex hypospadias, intersexualism) or traumas, essentially with a view to obtain an acceptable erectile function. However, the experimental prerequisites are not available yet, and the current risks of immune suppression probably exceed the potential benefits, because in such cases patients can usually have a normal or near normal social life. The particular case of transexualism, in its most disabling forms, may also be debated.

Our overall conclusion is that, in selected cases, CTAs have the potential to fill a gap in our therapeutic armamentarium against severely disabling conditions. In any case, whenever a given type of CTA appears medically and ethically acceptable, careful evaluation of its potential indications, using well-designed clinical trials, is mandatory before definite judgments can be made. Also, it should be kept in mind that, for CTAs as for other treatments, the balance between risks and benefits can shift one way or the other with time, depending in particular upon the progress of immune control of allotransplantation, and upon the progress of non-transplantation reconstructive or prosthetic techniques. Whether CTA techniques undergo a rapid development or not, the data gathered in the first clinical studies will be of paramount importance for future research as well as for future clinical trials.

Legal context for the procurement and grafting of organs and tissues: the French situation

Shortly summarised, the French legal frame, for the procurement and grafting of human organs or tissues from deceased donors is as follows (see also *Table I*):

1. For both tissues and organs, the institution where the harvesting procedure takes place must be officially authorised.

Table I. Essentials of the comparative legal status of tissues and organs

	Tissues	Organs	Comments
Harvesting only in authorised institutions	+	+	
Non-payment	+	+	
Anonymity	+	+	
Consent	+	+	
Therapeutic purpose	Presumed consent	Presumed consent	Includes clinical trials
Scientific purpose	Explicit consent	Explicit consent	
CMV, EBV, toxoplasmosis serology performed in donor	Not mandatory	Mandatory	Additional safety information for immunosuppressed recipients
Allografts performed only in authorised institutions	No	Yes	Tissues grafted in any public or private surgical facility, whereas organs grafted in teaching public hospitals only

2. For both tissues and organs, a number of mandatory tests must be performed in the donor for safety reasons. In the case of organs, three additional tests are mandatory, *i.e.* cytomegalovirus, Epstein-Barr virus and toxoplasmosis serology.

3. For organs only, the institution where the grafting takes place must have been specifically authorised and is mandatorily a teaching public hospital or a university-affiliated public structure.

4. For both organs and tissues, three general principles are the foundation of allograft procurement: non-payment (to the donor or donor relatives), reciprocal anonymity of donor and recipient, donor consent.

5. In terms of consent to organ, tissue or cell donation from deceased potential donors, since 1994 the French legislation considers two specific situations. The retrieval may be planned with a "therapeutic purpose", and is then legally possible if the deceased had not formerly expressed his or her opposition to the donation. This situation is associated with the notion of "presumed" or "implicit" consent. Conversely, the retrieval may be planned with a "scientific purpose", and is then legally possible only if the deceased had formerly expressed his positive will to donate. This situation is associated with the notion of "explicit consent". In both cases, the knowledge of the will of the deceased is obtained, among other procedures (mandatory interrogation of the National Registry of Refusals), by an inquiry among the relatives or next of kin of the deceased, who are invited to testify about the will of the deceased.

The applicable regimen for CTAs is therefore that of presumed consent to donate, since there is an obvious and direct therapeutic purpose. The fact that some CTAs are performed within a clinical trial has no effect on this situation.

Legal status of CTAs

The question of whether the legal status of CTAs is that of tissues or that of organs, or is neither of those is therefore relevant, because defining the legal status of CTAs has administrative, judicial, and practical consequences.

The French laws and regulations refer to only three types of grafts: cells, organs or tissues. The precise definition of tissues and organs is otherwise taken for granted, and it is usually understood that the term "organ" designates the liver, kidney, heart, lung, intestine or pancreas. An explicit additional definition states that bone marrow is considered to be an organ. At present in France, the legal and regulatory status of CTAs is not defined, since CTAs themselves are neither defined nor even considered by the current regulations. However, it is apparent that most technical characteristics of CTAs render them extremely similar to organ allografts, as shown in *Table II*. These features are:

1. Donors must be heart-beating donors.
2. The quality of the graft may be influenced by the resuscitation history of the donor.
3. The duration of conservation of the graft, once harvested, is short (storage for later use is not possible).
4. The ischemia time of the graft is likely to influence the vitality of the graft, its immunological acceptance, and the final functional result.
5. Living, immunogenic donor cells are grafted, and have to survive in contact with the recipient's blood and immune system.
6. Immunosuppression is therefore mandatory, although there have been examples where immunosuppression was only temporarily needed (joints, flexor systems, nerves) and, in some cases, may need to be stronger than for most visceral organ grafts.

Table II. "Organ-like" features of CTAs

	Tissues	Organs	CTAs
Heart-beating donors	+	+	+
Non heart-beating donors	+	No	No
Influence of resuscitation history	±	+++	++?
Storage possible	In most cases	No	No
Deleterious effect of ischemia time	± or No	+++	+++
Immunogenic graft	Usually No	Yes	Yes
Living cells grafted	Usually No	Yes	Yes
Immunosuppression	Usually No	Yes	Usually Yes
Physico-chemical procedures to reduce infectious risks	Often possible	No	No
Need for waiting list/allocation rules	Cornea only	Yes	Yes in future

7. Procedures of bacterial or viral inactivation, as routinely performed for some non-vascularised tissue grafts, cannot be used.

8. Suitable potential donors are few, due to the mutilating character of the retrieval as well as to the stringent donor selection criteria (for instance age, sex, morphology, in addition to blood group and possibly MHC antigens). If CTAs become more common, it will then become necessary to set up a waiting list and to define allocation rules, as for visceral organs today.

Conversely, essentially because of the variety and heterogeneous nature of the grafts, the term CTA has been coined which describes adequately the technical nature of such grafts.

In practical terms, in order to manage the current situation, it was chosen not to define CTAs as organ grafts, thus avoiding the need for a lengthy administrative procedure of authorisation of the site of surgery, and the need for a waiting list. This does not mean that any CTA can be performed anywhere on any patient since, at this stage, clinical trials of CTAs must be declared to the national Health Products Safety Agency (AFSSAPS) and can be vetoed by the Minister of Health.

For all other technical aspects, in particular concerning donor screening, it was decided to organise CTAs in the same way as organ grafts, albeit with a number of specificities owing to the nature of the retrieved anatomical parts.

It is likely that, if CTAs become more commonly performed, a specific legal status will have to be defined to accommodate this new type of graft, and it is likely that this status will be closer to that of organs than to that of tissues, in order to guarantee that only competent, well-structured multidisciplinary teams embark on such complex surgical, medical and paramedical procedures.

CTAs specificity with regard to fundamental principles of donation in France (non-payment, consent, anonymity)

1. Non-payment: the principle of non-payment is applicable without particular problems to the case of CTAs.

2. Consent: because the retrieval of the composite tissue allograft may affect visible parts of the body, such as hands or forearms, it may have a deep psychological impact on the process of grieving in relatives. It is therefore paramount that the exact nature of the retrieval should be explained to the relatives, as well as the technique of body restoration. In fact, the applicable regimen of "presumed consent" may not be totally adequate in some cases, and in practice it is advisable to proceed only if it is clear that the relatives themselves have been fully informed of, have understood, and do not disagree with the procedure.

3. Donor-recipient anonymity: according to article L. 1211-5. of the Code of Public Health, *"the donor should not know the recipient's identity, and the recipient should not know the donor's identity. No piece of information allowing the simultaneous identification of both the person having donated part of or a product of his/her body and* *of the person who received it should be divulged. Derogation is possible only in case of therapeutic necessity".*

In the case of CTAs, there is no therapeutic necessity to justify a breach of the anonymity principle. The anonymity of the donor can usually be protected, although one must be extremely cautious on this point within the procurement hospital. Conversely, for the most dramatic procedures (larynx, hands...), due to the intensive media coverage which usually takes place, it is illusory to try and maintain the anonymity of the recipient. It is even likely that the donor's relatives will see pictures of the recipient, and possibly of body parts of their deceased donor. Because this may cause great distress, it is of paramount importance that these issues should be discussed beforehand with the donor's family. Also, it is necessary to emphasize that despite this possible one-way breach of anonymity, no relationship should be set up between the recipient(s) and the donor's family.

Body restoration

According to article L. 1232-5 of the Code of Public Health, *"the physicians having performed retrieval (of an organ) from a deceased person have to ensure the decent restoration of his/her body".*

Also, Good Practice Guidelines indicate with some more details the way the body must be "decently restored" before being handed back to the bereaved relatives after retrieval of organs or tissues [16, 17]. Although the particular case of the various possibilities of CTAs is not explicitly detailed in these guidelines, common sense and sympathy with the relatives should prove sufficient for the surgical team to find the best possible solution. In all cases, the techniques used should have been prepared (and, if necessary, tested) well beforehand, discussed with the retrieval team, and the final result should be explained to the relatives with sufficient detail so as to avoid misunderstandings and potential conflicts. Also, depending upon the specificity of each case, it is probably wise to limit retrievals for CTAs in a given donor, in spite of the rarity of suitable donors. It may otherwise be impossible to ensure a "decent" body restoration.

Potential effects of hand allograft procurement on the general level of organ donation

Because of the rather dramatic nature and high media coverage of hand allografts, fears have been expressed that they might have a negative effect on the rate of organ donation in France. The follow-up of the organ donation rate in France *(Figure 1)* has shown that:

1. the organ procurement rate in France is, expectedly, variable with time. Between 1993 and 2001, the monthly number of deceased organ donors has commonly varied between 65 and 90, with occasional troughs as low as 45 and peaks as high as 105 donors. In spite of that, the yearly number of donors does not show any dramatic trend *(Figure 1)*;

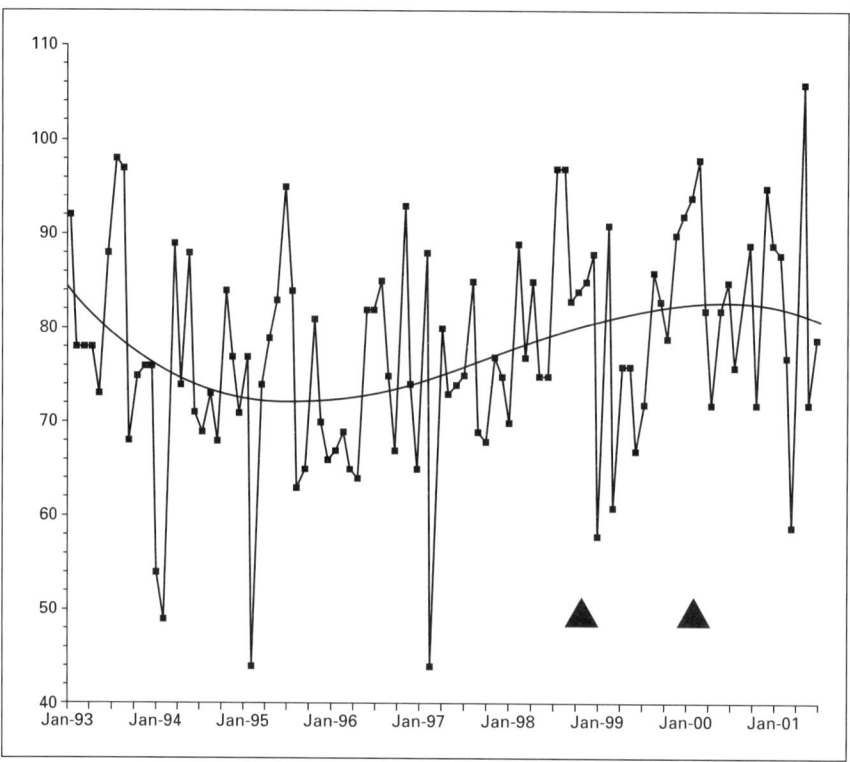

Figure 1. Monthly number of organ donors, France, 1993-2001. ■ Monthly number of donors; — Cubic regression; ▲ Date of hand allografts (France).

2. since 1993, there has been some degree of yearly periodicity in the national monthly number of donors, with a clear trough at the beginning of the year, for as yet unclear and probably multifactorial reasons *(Figure 1)*;

3. no statistically significant positive or negative anomaly of the organ donation rate has been observed at the national level in the months following the two hand allografts in France *(Figure 1)*.

Donor rates in the Eastern central area of France (inter-region number 3 as defined by the Etablissement français des Greffes), where the hand allografts were performed, were also analysed. The data do not suggest any clear positive or negative impact of the hand allograft procedures *(Figure 2)*.

In spite of these reassuring figures, it should not be assumed that dramatic procedures such as hand allografts cannot have negative consequences on organ donation, and we should always remain extremely cautious in our approach of the donor families, of the media and of the general public.

It should also be kept in mind that the professional community at large may react to some CTAs in an unfavourable way, some specialists expressing more or less publicly their disagreement with the procedures performed, as is natural and even desirable in

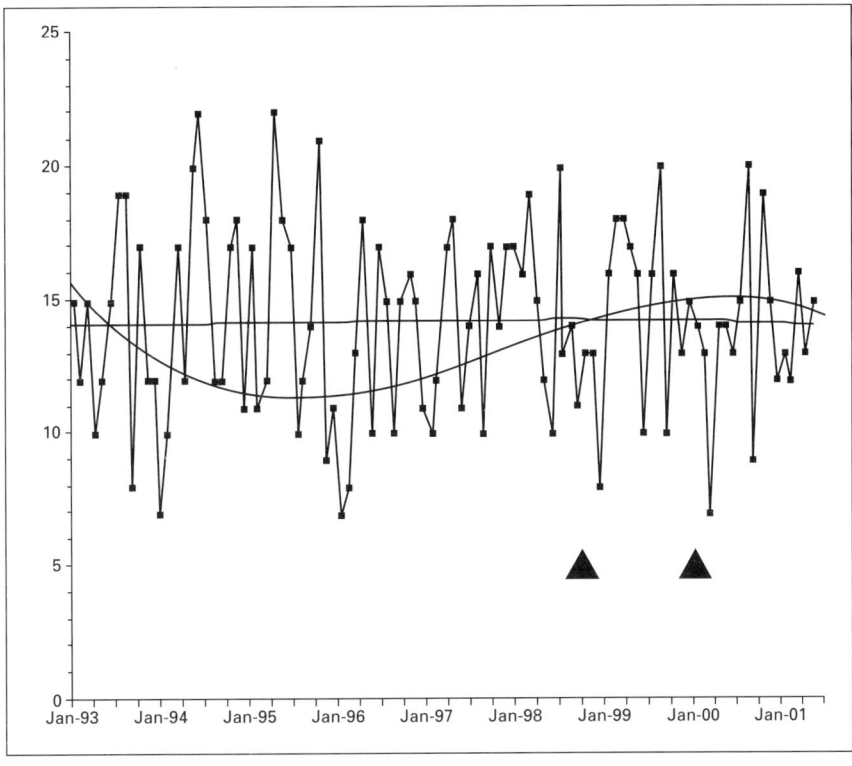

Figure 2. Monthly number of organ donors, Eastern central area of France, 1993-2001. ■ Monthly number of donors; — Cubic regression; ▲ Date of hand allografts (France).

a democratic environment. Such debate is indeed inevitable because we are dealing with therapeutic research, where controversy is the rule rather than the exception. However, we believe that overheated public debates or extreme positions should be avoided in the profession, because they may create diffidence in the public against the whole activity of transplantation in general, with negative effects on the patients at large.

Conclusion

CTAs are a promising therapeutic research area, for which the first clinical applications are now being investigated. CTAs demand a specific approach of the donation act, essentially due to the unusual character of the body parts harvested, to the potentially strong psychological impact of the retrieval procedure, and to the possibly excessive media coverage.

Because CTAs are sophisticated, aggressive therapeutic techniques still in the realm of clinical research, some degree of controversy among professionals is both inevitable and necessary. However, the community should be protected from the possible consequences of publicised overreactions which might create, *via* biased media coverage, suspicion against CTAs and even against the transplantation activity in general, resulting in a decreased rate of organ and tissue donation, and ultimately in undue patient deaths. In our view, the only way to avoid such a regrettable chain of events is to proceed with CTAs at a reasonable pace, openly, using well-structured evaluation procedures in well-designed clinical trials, after in-depth review of the proposed trials by the appropriate regulatory, scientific and ethical authorities. It is with this philosophy in mind that the current bilateral hand allograft clinical trial programme has been designed in France.

References

1. Llull R. An open proposal for clinical composite tissue allotransplantation. *Transplant Proc* 1998; 30: 2692-6.
2. Hewitt CW. Update and outline of the experimental problems facing clinical composite tissue transplantation. *Transplant Proc* 1998; 30: 2704-7.
3. Hofmann GO, Kirschner MH, Wagner FD, Brauns L, Gonschorek O, Bühren V. Allogeneic vascularized transplantation of human femoral diaphyses and total knee joints – First clinical experiences. *Transplant Proc* 1998; 30: 2754-61.
4. Jones TR, Humphrey PA, Brennan DC. Transplantation of vascularized allogeneic skeletal muscle for scalp reconstruction in a renal transplant patient. *Transplant Proc* 1998; 30: 2746-53.
5. Bain JR. Peripheral nerve allografting: review of the literature with relevance to composite tissue transplantation. *Transplant Proc* 1998; 30: 2762-7.
6. Guimberteau JC, Baudet J, Panconi B, Boileau R, Potaux I. Human allotransplant of a complete digital flexion system vascularized on the ulnar pedicle: a preliminary report and 1-year follow-up of two cases. *Plastic Reconstr Surg* 1992; 89: 1135-47.
7. Dubernard JM, Owen E, Guillaume Herzberg G, Lanzetta M, Martin X, Kapila H, Dawahra M, Hakim NS. Human hand allograft: report on first 6 months. *Lancet* 1999; 353: 1315-20.
8. Kanitakis J, Jullien D, Claudy A, Revillard JP, Dubernard JM. Microchimerism in a human hand allograft. *Lancet* 1999; 354: 1820-1.
9. Kanitakis J, Jullien D, De Boer B, Claudy A, Dubernard JM. Regeneration of cutaneous innervation in a human hand allograft. *Lancet* 2000; 356: 1738-9.
10. Kanitakis J, Jullien D, Nicolas JF, Frances C, Claudy A, Revillard JP, Owen E, Dubernard JM. Sequential histological and immunohistochemical study of the skin of the first human hand allograft. *Transplantation* 2000; 69: 1380-5.
11. Kanitakis J, Jullien D, Petruzzo P, Frances C, Claudy A, Revillard JP, Dubernard JM. Immunohistologic Studies of the skin of human hand allografts: our experience with two patients. *Transplant Proc* 2001; 33: 1722.
12. Giraux P, Sirigu A, Schneider F, Dubernard JM. Cortical reorganization in motor cortex after graft of both hands. *Nat Neurosci* 2001; 4: 691-2.
13. Jones JW, Gruber SA, Barker JH, Breidenbach WC. Successful hand transplantation, one-year follow-up. *N Engl J Med* 2000; 343: 468-73.
14. François CG, Breidenbach WC, Maldonado C, Kakoulidis TP, Hodges A, Dubernard JM, Owen E, Pei G, Ren X, Barker JH. Hand transplantation: comparisons and observations of the first four clinical cases. *Microsurgery* 2000; 20: 360-71.
15. Strome M, Stein J, Esclamado R, Hicks D, Lorenz RR, Braun W, Yetman R, Eliachar I, Mayes J. Laryngeal transplantation and 40-month follow-up. *N Engl J Med* 2001; 344: 1676-9.
16. Arrêté du 27 février 1998 portant homologation des règles de bonnes pratiques relatives au prélèvement d'organes à finalité thérapeutique sur personne décédée. *Journal Officiel de la République Française*, numéro 73 du 27 mars 1998, p. 4625.
17. Arrêté du 1er avril 1997 portant homologation des règles de bonnes pratiques relatives au prélèvement de tissus à finalité thérapeutique sur personne décédée. *Journal Officiel de la République Française*, numéro 81 du 6 avril 1997, p. 5275.

Ethical arguments in favor and against the composite tissue allografts

Didier Sicard
Service de Médecine interne, CHU Cochin, Paris, France

An ethical discussion is preferable to an ethical judgment given prior to taking action. It is more advisable not to submit in advance medical or surgical protocols based on an arbitrary moral determination, acting as if the problem was already resolved by transcendental references (and what references?). This is even more true given that medical science is never satisfactorily based on the past and incurs as much hopes as fears which are more or less justified.

With respect to the composite tissue allografts (CTA), four issues can be raised:

1. If at first we had to fight against the oppositions to organs, kidney and even hearts grafts, these oppositions are now overcome. But is it possible to ethically think that the current ordinariness of these organ grafts will be – with time – considered as ordinary for the CTA?

2. Shall we have a conservative or liberal reasoning?

3. Should therapeutic performance have priority over the principle of well-being?

4. Is it possible to assimilate the CTA with usual clinical research?

Dealing with those four issues, we find four tentative answers which are rather on the negative side.

1. No comparison is made possible since those grafts do not deal with the substantial mechanisms of life.

2. Liberalism can be as dynamic as it can be adventurous, conservatism can be as cautionary as it can be apprehensive.

3. Therapeutic performance only as a goal is not ethical.

4. The CTA are not part of the usual clinical research.

The ethical discussion should take place, knowing that this is not going to be a match, with a winner and a loser, but the outcome of which should leave us better informed.

Rather than having arguments in favor or against something, which would give the impression of leaning to one side or another, we should raise questions, knowing that it is always dangerous to ask for an ethical judgment after the fact, like an endorsement of an accomplished fact.

It would be like having in successive steps: the desire, the project, the research and animal experimentation, the writing of the protocol, the surgery and then lastly the ethical reflection. A sort of "post" ethics?

I will center the discussion on the CTA related to body parts grafts.

1. **Contributing to the well-being of individuals is a principle which is at the very core of all medical acts**. In this particular context, is this principle being contradicted by a negative principle or is it just a balance between benefits and negative risks?

The desire of a wounded individual to be cured is legitimate but his/her hope to have his/her body back as well as its motions may sometimes be a goal for which he/she is ready to take vital risks. It is in those terms of choices that consent has to be asked, without omitting to tell such an individual that the vital risk does not necessarily result in a functional success, even if there is a possibility to recuperate a function compatible with a normal life. As opposed to organ grafts, the evolution of science – in terms of time – which will allow a more and more satisfactory functioning of body parts, will lead **to less and less acceptable** immunodepressive therapeutic constrainsts, and even more so because the hand has a conscious functioning based on will, unlike the liver, the heart and the kidney. The experiment of continuous therapies for the heart, kidney or liver grafts or for HIV infections show the psychological limit of tolerance when having to constantly use medicine. We cannot hide to young wounded individuals who will be going under surgery that they will receive a therapy for decades which will eventually **shorten their lives**, because of premature aging, an accelerated atherosclerosis, an infectious vulnerability, or maybe a lymphoma or melanoma. The issue is not one of a 5 but rather a 30 or 40 year period. Therefore, the principle to provide for the well-being of individuals has a counterpart of potential serious drawbacks (like the shortening of life). Thinking in terms of ordinariness for immunosuppressive treatments which are given in other types of illnesses or grafts may be considered more an opportunist measure than an ethical reflection and cannot allow the wounded person to express her/himself.

2. **Is it an innovative therapeutic performance which needs to be encouraged**?

Several arguments can be made:

– Certain people think that auto-grafts have been perfected and that in this surgical area the allograft does not teach anything more. They argue that the neuronal cortical reorganization capacity delay – because of a peripheral stimulation – is most unlikely, or that in any case, the capacity to do a voluntary movement coordinated from a cortical command is unlikely; even if we assume that "the hand makes the brain" and not the contrary, this reasoning cannot apply to a graft.

– However, on the opposite side, experimental studies have shown – with the functional IRM – that cortical areas can change along with the post-graft evolution and this unexpected information is encouraging.

– The core issue which remains is: are we dealing more with therapy or research or neither one? It is not therapy because it is not based on scientific certainty and it is not research because a non-validated therapeutic does not automatically constitute research.

But it is more a therapeutic performance whose natural effects are not small, whether in regard to skin grafts for burnt patients or for the physiology of nervous regeneration.

3. **Can a body part graft be integrated into the body scheme whether on a short term or long term basis**? The identity of a composite tissue donor cannot invade the identity of a receiver, except in movies ("Les mains d'Orlac" from R. Wiene 1933, and E. T. Greville 1950), but the permanent visibility of what is the most intimate, the most in contact with the other, the most affectionate (we hold the hand of a dying person) may create a severe schizoidy. Integration or disintegration are not issues which are raised with other organ grafts or other composite tissues. Here, the receiver, who slowly realizes that it is not his/her hand, may experience a conflicting situation that he/she would not experience with a mechanical prosthesis. It is true that in this domain, research remains to be done, our ignorance is vast in terms of the human capacity to integrate "the strange foreigner". The tension between the physical aspect and the symbolic representation is maximal because of the hand's role in the economy of our organism.

4. **The problem of the anonymous aspect of grafts, besides living donors, is a substantial principle**. Here, it is eliminated for the receiver and also, sometimes, for the donor. Recently a receiver was thanking the family of a murderer who had committed suicide. The risk of dealing with morbid curiosity, investigation by the donor's family into the identity of the receiver of the hand cannot be excluded and may be at the source of fantasies which are so much more important: that hand has a story. It would be tempting to choose body parts from isolated individuals with no families but such specific research would raise major ethical issues.

5. **Can the consent of a donor be implied or expressed in such a situation**? Inasmuch as it is acceptable for most human beings to consent to donate their liver, heart, etc. it is much more complex in our imagination to donate an arm or specifically a hand or two hands. In the case of a composite tissue graft surgery, it is important to integrate this dimension right now in the questionnaires given to potential future donors.

6. **The composite tissue grafts also raise the issue of an indefinitely reparable human body**. This **functionalist**, rational, mechanical vision is being very exclusive and rejects everything that is not functional. **Ethics are here to remind us that life is not only about functionality**, ethics is resisting with tenacity to functionality, as our humanity should require, as we do not belong to ourselves, as self-respect cannot be separated from respect to others, to the body, to its integrity and its unity.

Therefore, if composite tissue grafts constitute an undeniable benefit for a large number of tissues, tendons, skin, cartilage, bones, etc. the issue of the hand, or the arm, or the leg graft is still raised. Of course the desire to recuperate a function, the quality of surgery teams, the research whether experimental or not, will give arguments in favor of continuing and encouraging this type of activity but the ethical reflection implies that the reflection on the human being be not limited to the technical success of surgery even when it is spectacular.

Aknowledgements: Many thanks to Oriane Shevin and Ann Atik in helping to translate.

Lecture

Composite Tissue Allografts
Dubernard J.-M., ed.
© John Libbey Eurotext, Paris, 2001

Composite tissue allografts: perspectives from a laboratory

W.P. Andrew Lee, David W. Mathes, Mark A. Randolph, Peter E.M. Butler
Plastic Surgery Research Laboratory, Massachusetts General Hospital, Harvard Medical School, Boston, Massachusetts, USA

At least nine hand transplants have been performed in the world since 1998. Is hand transplantation a breakthrough that will flourish in the 21st century? Or is it "technology over good sense"? As with any surgery recommended to our patients, we must consider and balance its feasible benefits, likelihood of success based on current knowledge and scientific data, and potential complications [1]. Each of these points will be examined here from the perspective of a laboratory that has engaged in research of composite tissue allografts for nearly two decades.

With the advent of microvascular surgery, transplantation of composite tissue allografts has long been technically feasible consisting of any combination of skin, subcutaneous tissue, nerve, blood vessel, muscle, bone, or the whole limb. Patients who can benefit from composite tissue transplants include not just traumatic amputees, but those with congenital deformities and those requiring reconstruction after tumor resection, where current modalities are inadequate such as frozen bone allografts. Even patients with facial disfigurement stand to benefit from transplants of body parts. Thus the feasible benefits of composite tissue allografts are immense by allowing customized reconstruction with vascularized tissues that have theoretically an unlimited supply and leave no donor site morbidity.

Much work has been done in animal models to study host rejection of limb allografts. Unlike organ allografts with largely homogeneous tissues, a limb allograft consists of many tissue components. In our laboratory, we developed rat models of transplantation for *each* individual tissue component of a limb allograft: skin, subcutaneous tissue, muscle, bone, blood vessels, and the entire hind limb [2]. After transplant, host spleen cells were harvested and grown in a mixed lymphocyte culture to measure the cell-mediated immune response. Host serum was collected upon sacrifice and assayed with complements for antibodies to measure the humoral immune response. We found that muscle elicited the most intense responses at both 1 and 2 weeks after transplant. Skin, subcutaneous tissue, and bone were about equally antigenic. The limb allografts, consisting of all the tissue components, generated surprisingly lower responses, possibly representing a "consumption" phenomenon. The pattern for humoral responses was different in that muscle allografts generated no antibody production until 2 weeks. The humoral response to limb allografts was lower at 1 week, but similar to other tissues at 2 weeks. Thus there is a hierarchy of antigenicity for limb tissue components, that varies according to the type of immune response measured and the time it was measured. Rejection of limb allografts, therefore, appears far more complex than that of organ allografts.

It is not surprising, then, that experimental composite tissue transplantation have met with mixed results. The findings in different animal models will be briefly summarized. In the rats, cyclosporine alone did not prevent rejection of limb allograft in most animals except when given at toxic doses [3, 4]. FK-506 was found to be more effective in preventing rejection, but animals frequently developed *Pneumocystis carinii* pneumonia [5]. Combination therapy using low dose cyclosporine and mycophenolate was able to achieve prolonged survival without significant toxicity [6]. The primate data were discouraging. Despite high-dose cyclosporine and steroids in three studies, very few limb transplants survived to 300 days, and many animals died from complications [7, 8]. The Louisville group transplanted osteomyocutaneous flaps from the radial forelimb of outbred swine. The recipient animals received prednisone, mycophenolate, and either cyclosporine or FK-506. About a third of the animals showed no evidence of rejection at 90 days [9].

In our laboratory, we have aimed to achieve limb transplantation without long-term immunosuppression. The MGH (Massachusetts General Hospital) miniature swine was used, which are the only large animal species with defined major histocompatibility complex (MHC) allowing the study of different transplantation barriers between donor and recipient. For example, transplants between siblings with the same haplotypes can be simulated by swine with MHC match and only minor antigen differences. In our experimental model, an allograft consisting of tibia, fibula, and distal femur with surrounding muscles based on the femoral vascular pedicle was transplanted [10]. The vascular pedicle was anastomosed to the recipient femoral vessels, and the graft secured in a subcutaneous pocket in the abdominal wall. All allografts with complete MHC mismatch and 12 days of cyclosporine treatment were rejected by 42 days. Allografts with MHC match and only minor antigen differences not treated with cyclosporine showed rejection between 63 and 84 days. Allografts with minor antigen differences and 12 days of cyclosporine were still alive at harvest between 178 and 280 days as evident by gross inspection and histologic sections [11]. Swine tolerant of limb tissue allografts received freeze-preserved donor skin grafts and third-party control skin grafts to confirm systemic tolerance. Third party control skin grafts were rejected between 8 and 13 days, while skin grafts from the limb donor showed significantly prolonged survival (48 to 100 days), thus confirming specific tolerance to the limb donor while maintaining immune competence. To investigate the degree of chimerism in the recipient animals, a non-MHC marker pig allelic antigen (PAA) was used in transplants performed from PAA+ donor to PAA- recipient. We found that the peripheral chimerism was as high as 2% initially after the transplant, but completely dissipated about a week after cessation of cyclosporine, despite acceptance of the graft without rejection [12]. The donor cells in the graft marrow also steadily dissipated with time, thus providing evidence for the process of creeping substitution by recipient cells [13]. Thus tolerance to musculo-skeletal allografts (without skin) can be induced in miniature swine with minor antigen differences using a short course of cyclosporine. Clinically, genetic matching does not apply to just family members, as the National Bone Marrow Registry exists to match unrelated individuals.

According to our experimental data, genetic matching can significantly alter the risk-benefit balance of composite tissue transplantation by eliminating the reliance on chronic immunosuppression with its concomitant adverse effects. Toxicity of immunosuppressants such as nephrotoxicity and onset of diabetes is well established [14, 15]. In published studies, 88% of organ transplant recipients develop at least one episode of opportunistic infection [16]. There is a 4 to 18% chance of developing malignancies, most commonly squamous cell carcinoma of skin and lymphoma [17, 18]. Since composite tissue transplant increases the quality but not the quantity of life, it is our opinion that future composite tissue transplant depends upon reducing or even eliminating the need for long-term immunosuppression [19].

Other than immunosuppression and genetic matching, tolerance induction represents another strategy for achieving transplantation of any organ or tissues [20]. In our laboratory, we have attempted to induce tolerance to composite tissue allografts by marrow injection into the thymus, by marrow injection immediately after birth into a peripheral vein, and by marrow injection into the fetal portal circulation.

In the thymic experiment, bone marrow cells from Brown-Norway rats were harvested from the long bones and injected into the thymus of young Lewis recipients. The Lewis rats then underwent transplantation of a full thickness skin graft from BN rats. Animals receiving intrathymic bone marrow showed more than a three time prolongation in survival time over the control allograft [21]. In the neonatal experiment, we utilized Medawar's finding half a century ago in inducing tolerance to skin graft by exposure to donor antigen in the neonatal mice. Bone marrow cells were harvested from the long bones of Brown Norway rats. Neonatal Lewis rats within 12 hours of birth were injected with the marrow suspension into the temporal vein under magnification. A heterotopic musculoskeletal knee allograft was then performed. All isografts survived, while all allografts into untreated Lewis rats were rejected. Two-thirds of the Lewis rats injected with Brown Norway marrow accepted the allografts without rejection [22].

Most recently, we utilized Owen's observation in 1945 that placental exchange of hematopoietic cells between dizygotic cattle twins led to life-long tolerance of each other's tissue despite genetic differences. In our experiment, boar and sow were screened before mating to ensure strong response to the donor. At mid-gestation the donor marrow was harvested and depleted of T-cells using antibodies conjugated with magnetic beads. A laparotomy was performed in the pregnant sow to expose the uterus. The fetuses were identified using ultrasound, and the marrow suspension was injected into the portal circulation of individual fetal swine. Following birth of the piglets, *in vitro* and *in vivo* testing were conducted [23]. A clear population of chimeric cells were noted in the chimeric piglet by FACS analysis, while some of its litter mates demonstrated none. Mixed lymphocyte reactions showed a clear difference between the strong anti-donor response in the non-chimeric piglets and the low response by the chimeric piglets. In the cell-mediated lysis assay, all piglets reacted strongly to a third party control, whereas the chimeric piglets demonstrated no response against the donor. *In vivo* tolerance was tested using skin grafts from the piglet itself, donor, matched third party, and unmatched third party. In the non-chimeric piglet, all but the autologous skin grafts were rejected. In the chimeric piglets, *in vivo* tolerance was demonstrated by acceptance of the donor and matched third party skin graft and rejection of the unmatched skin graft with complete healing by 22 days. Humoral assays after skin grafts showed emergence of anti-donor antibodies in the non-chimeric piglets, but none in the tolerant piglets [24].

In order to confirm donor specific tolerance, the chimeric swine accepted donor-matched kidney allografts with a stable creatinine until sacrifice more than 300 days after transplant [24, 25]. When the more antigenic composite tissue allografts were transplanted in a heterotopic musculoskeletal model as described above, the chimeric swine also exhibited tolerance without evidence of rejection until sacrifice up to 242 days in four animal [26].

To summarize, composite tissue transplantation offers immense potential, but its risk-benefit balance must be carefully weighed [27]. Alteration of this balance by reducing or even eliminating immunosuppression would facilitate widespread clinical application of these allografts. Such is the goal of a laboratory long engaged in the research of composite tissue transplantation.

References

1. Lee WPA, Mathes DW. Hand transplantation: pertinent data and future outlook. *J Hand Surg* 1999; 24A: 906-13.
2. Lee WPA, Yaremchuk MJ, Pan YC, Randolph MA, Tan CM, Weiland AJ. Relative antigenicity of components of a vascularized limb allograft. *Plast Reconstr Surg* 1991; 87: 401-11.
3. Black KS, Hewitt CW, Hwang JS, *et al.* Dose response of cyclosporine-treated composite tissue allografts in a strong histoincompatible rat model. *Transplant Proc* 1988; 20 (2 Suppl. 2): 266-8.
4. Lee WPA, Pan YC, Kesmarky S, Randolph MA, Fiala TS, Amarante MTJ, Weiland AJ, Yaremchuk MJ. Experimental orthotopic transplantation of vascularized skeletal allografts: functional assessment and long-term survival. *Plast Reconstr Surg* 1995; 95: 336-49.
5. Buttemeyer R, Jones NF, Min Z, Rao U. Rejection of the component tissues of limb allografts in rats immunosuppressed with FK-506 and cyclosporine. *Plast Reconstr Surg* 1996; 97: 139-48; discussion 149-51.
6. Benhaim P, Anthony JP, Ferreira L, *et al.* Use of combination of low-dose cyclosporine and RS-61443 in a rat hindlimb model of composite tissue allotransplantation. *Transplantation* 1996; 61: 527-32.
7. Daniel RK, Egerszegi EP, Samulack DD, *et al.* Tissue transplants in primates for upper extremity reconstruction: a preliminary report. *J Hand Surg [Am]* 1986; 11(1): 1-8.
8. Stark GB, Swartz WM, Narayanan K, Moller AR. Hand transplantation in baboons. *Transplant Proc* 1987; 19: 3968-71.
9. Ustuner ET, Zdichavsky M, Ren X, *et al.* Long-term composite tissue allograft survival in a porcine model with cyclosporine/mycophenolate mofetil therapy. *Transplantation* 1998; 66: 1581-7.
10. Lee WPA, Rubin JP, Cober S, Ierino F, Randolph MA, Sachs DH. Use Of swine model in transplantation of vascularized skeletal tissue allografts. *Transplant Proc* 1998; 30: 2743-945.
11. Lee WPA, Rubin JP, Bourget JL, Cober SR, Randolph MA, Nielsen GP, Ierino FL, Sachs DH. Tolerance to limb tissue allografts between swine matched for major histocompatibility complex antigens. *Plast Reconstr Surg* 2001; 107: 1482-90.
12. Bourget JL, Mathes DW, Nielsen GP, Randolph MA, Tanabe YN, Ferrara VR, Wu A, Arn S, Sachs DH, Lee WPA. Tolerance to musculoskeletal allografts with transient lymphocytic chimerism in miniature swine. *Transplantation* 2001; 71: 851-6.
13. Mathes DW, Bourget JL, Randolph MA, Sachs DH, Lee WPA. Recipient bone marrow engraftment in donor tissue following long-term tolerance to hemopoietic musculoskeletal allograft. *Plast Surg Forum* 1999; 22: 204-5.
14. Myers BD, Ross J, Newton L, *et al.* Cyclosporine-associated chronic nephropathy. *N Engl J Med* 1984; 311: 699-705.
15. Shapiro R, Fung JJ, Jain AB, *et al.* The side effects of FK 506 in humans. *Transplant Proc* 1990; 22: 35-6.

16. Dummer JS, Hardy A, Poorsattar A, Ho M. Early infections in kidney, heart, and liver transplant recipients on cyclosporine. *Transplantation* 1983; 36: 259-67.
17. Shaw LM, Kaplan B, Kaufman D. Toxic effects of immunosuppressive drugs: mechanisms and strategies for controlling them. *Clin Chem* 1996; 42: 1316-21.
18. Penn I. Malignancy. *Surg Clin North Am* 1994; 74: 1247-57.
19. Mathes DW, Lee WPA. Composite tissue transplantation: more science and patience needed. *Plast Reconstr Surg* 2001; 107: 1066-70.
20. Mathes DW, Randolph MA, Lee WPA. Strategies for tolerance induction to composite tissue allografts. *Microsurg* 2000; 20: 448-52.
21. Cober SR, Randolph MA, Lee WPA. Skin allograft survival following intrathymic injection of donor bone marrow. *J Surg Res* 1999; 85: 204-8.
22. Butler PEM, Lee WPA, Van de Water AP, Randolph MA. Neonatal induction of tolerance to skeletal tissue allografts without immunosuppression. *Plast Reconstr Surg* 2000; 105: 2424-30.
23. Rubin JP, Cober SR, Butler PEM, Randolph MA, Gazelle S, Ierino F, Sachs DH, Lee WPA. Injection of allogeneic bone marrow cells into the portal vein of swine *in utero*. *J Surg Res* 2001; 95: 188-94.
24. Mathes DW, Yamada K, Randolph MA, Utsugi R, Solari MG, Gazelle GS, Wu A, Sachs DH, Lee WPA. *In utero* induction of transplantation tolerance. *Transplant Proc* 2001; 33: 98-100.
25. Mathes DW, Yamada Y, Randolph MA, Solari MG, Wu A, Gazelle GS, Sachs DH, Lee WPA. In utero induction of transplantation tolerance. *Proc Plast Surg Res Council* 2000; 45: 93.
26. Mathes DW, Randolph MA, Butler PEM, Solari MG, Gazelle GS, Sachs DH, Lee WPA. Intravascular *in utero* injection of adult bone marrow leads to acceptance of fully mismatched composite tissue allografts. *Surg Forum* 2001, in press.
27. Hettiaratchy S, Butler PEM, Lee WPA. Lessons from hand transplantation. *Lancet* 2001; 357: 494-5.

Achevé d'imprimer par 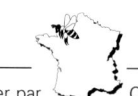 Corlet, Imprimeur, S.A.
14110 Condé-sur-Noireau (France)
N° d'Imprimeur : 3501 - Dépôt légal : novembre 2001
Imprimé en U.E.